The Anatomy and Physiology of Obstetrics

by the same author

*

A SUMMARY OF GYNAECOLOGY

THE FABER POCKET DICTIONARY OF MIDWIFERY

The Anatomy and Physiology of Obstetrics

A SHORT TEXTBOOK FOR STUDENTS AND MIDWIVES

C. W. F. BURNETT

M.D., F.R.C.S., F.R.C.O.G.

Obstetrician and Gynaecologist, West Middlesex Hospital; Gynaecologist, Staines Hospital; Vice-President of the Royal College of Midwives; Lecturer at the Midwife Teachers' Training College, Kingston-upon-Thames; Examiner to the Royal College of Obstetricians and Gynaecologists, The University of Khartoum, Sudan, the Central Midwives Board and General Nursing Council for England and Wales

WITH ILLUSTRATIONS BY

SUSAN ROBINSON, M.M.A.A.

Medical Artist, West Middlesex Hospital

FABER AND FABER

3 Queen Square

London

First published in 1953
by Faber and Faber Limited
3 Queen Square London WC1
Second edition 1959
Third edition 1962
Fourth edition 1965
Reprinted 1966
Fifth edition 1969
Reprinted 1971, 1972
Printed in Great Britain by
Latimer Trend & Company Ltd Plymouth

ISBN 0 571 04682 7 (hard-bound edition)

ISBN 0 571 09236 5 (paper covers)

Preface

In discussing maternity cases with medical students and midwives, and in examining candidates for the State Certificate and Teacher's Diploma of the Central Midwives Board, I have noticed that the subjects least understood and most disliked are the anatomy and physiology of the pelvis and the development of the fertilized ovum. Whilst this is unfortunate, because these form a necessary basis for the study of midwifery, it is at the same time quite intelligible, for their complete understanding can only be attained by dissecting the pelvic organs, performing physiological experiments and observing developmental processes. These are beyond the reach of most midwives and pupils, and this book has been written in an attempt to remedy the deficiency. Enough details are given to provide a comprehensive knowledge of these subjects, and I have endeavoured to rob them of their difficulties and to make them interesting rather than a mere succession of unrelated facts and figures.

It is hoped the book will enable practising midwives to keep their theoretical knowledge up to date; it is also designed to help candidates to learn the anatomy and physiology that are required for their qualifying examinations in midwifery. It should in addition prove of value to physiotherapists and radiographers and all those medical workers whose duties are concerned with the welfare of pregnant patients, and who therefore require some obstetrical knowledge. Chapter 2 is intended primarily for medical students and student teachers taking the Midwife Teacher's Diploma.

My thanks are due to Miss Susan Robinson for her drawings and illustrations. I am also indebted to Miss M. Gatenby, M.B.E., S.R.N., S.C.M., Miss M. Jones, S.R.N., S.C.M., M.T.D. and Miss D. Turner, S.R.N., S.C.M., M.T.D., who have each read the text and have offered many helpful criticisms. Special appreciation must be accorded to Mr. du Sautoy of Messrs. Faber & Faber Ltd., whose help and advice have at all times been placed freely at my disposal.

C. W. F. BURNETT

Department of Obstetrics,
West Middlesex Hospital,
Isleworth, Middlesex. March, 1953

Preface to Fifth Edition

It might be thought that subjects like anatomy and physiology would remain static and unchanged with the passage of time, but in recasting this present edition I have found that the advances in knowledge established during the last four years have necessitated many changes in the text. In our understanding of sex hormones in particular progress is continuously being made and this I have tried to record and describe.

Many of my readers have asked for new material or a changed format to be incorporated into the subject matter; I am grateful to them for their suggestions, which have all been carefully considered whether or not they have been adopted. I must thank Miss M. E. McKivett, S.R.N., S.C.M., M.T.D., D.N., of the Royal College of Midwives, at whose suggestion I have added a new Appendix dealing with cell life including the normal and abnormal forms of cell division. This is intended primarily for medical students and student midwife teachers.

I would like to pay a special tribute to Miss P. J. Cunningham, B.A., S.R.N., S.C.M., H.V.Cert., whose encouragement and advice during the preparation of this edition as in the past have proved invaluable.

C. W. F. BURNETT

November, 1968

Contents

Contents

Illustrations

CHAPTER 1

The Anatomy of the Female Genital Organs

The female genital organs are made up of the external genitalia, which comprise the structures of the vulva, and the internal genitalia, which include the vagina, uterus, Fallopian tubes and ovaries. These may together be said to form the female genital tract.

THE VULVA

The vulva is formed from the following structures:

(a) *The mons veneris* is a pad of fatty tissue situated in front of the symphysis pubis, covered by skin and pubic hairs which develop at the time of puberty. The hair is short and of the same colour as the hair of the scalp, with a typical distribution extending about one-third of the distance up to the umbilicus. Occasionally it reaches as high as this structure and then has the distribution which occurs normally in the male.

(b) *The labia majora* (each of which is known in the singular as a labium majus) consist of two rounded folds of fatty tissue and skin, which extend downwards and backwards from the mons veneris, enclosing between them the urogenital cleft. As they pass towards the anus they become flatter and merge into the perineal body, which lies between the lower end of the vagina in front and the anal canal behind. Their outer surface is covered with short hairs after puberty, whilst their inner surface is smooth and contains numerous sweat and sebaceous glands. The terminal portions of the round ligaments of the uterus end in the fatty tissues of the labia majora.

(c) *The labia minora* (which are known in the singular as a labium minus) are two smaller folds of pink skin lying longitudinally within the encircling labia majora and enclosing between them the vestibule.

They are quite smooth and devoid of hairs and fat, but they contain a few sweat and sebaceous glands and are very vascular.

When traced upwards and forwards each labium minus is seen to split into two smaller folds. The upper one of these unites with its fellow of the opposite side and forms the hood or prepuce of the clitoris; the smaller lower fold also joins with its fellow of the opposite side and both become attached to the under surface of the clitoris, where they form the frenulum of the clitoris. Thus the upper and

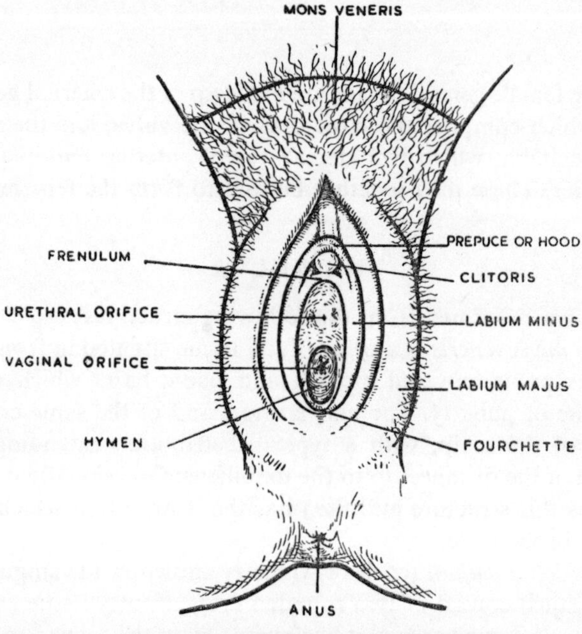

FIGURE 1. Diagram of the vulva

lower folds enclose the clitoris between them, with the prepuce lying above and the frenulum below.

When traced downwards and backwards the labia minora encircle the vagina and become joined together at their posterior extremities by a thin fold of skin known as the fourchette. It is this fold which is usually torn at the time of the patient's first delivery, however expert the midwife may be in controlling the birth of the baby's head.

(d) *The clitoris* is a small extremely sensitive erectile structure situated in the midline within the preputial and frenular folds of the labia minora. It is about one inch long and is composed of two corpora cavernosa, which are small erectile bodies lying side by side and extending backwards to be attached on each side to the underlying bones of the pubic arch. These portions are known as the crura (crus in the singular) of the clitoris. The pointed extremity of the clitoris or glans surmounts its body and is continuous with the vestibular bulbs presently to be described.

These structures are all extremely vascular with a plentiful nerve supply, and are attached by a small suspensory ligament to the front of the symphysis pubis. They correspond to similar structures which form the penis of the male, but are much smaller in size and do not transmit the urethra.

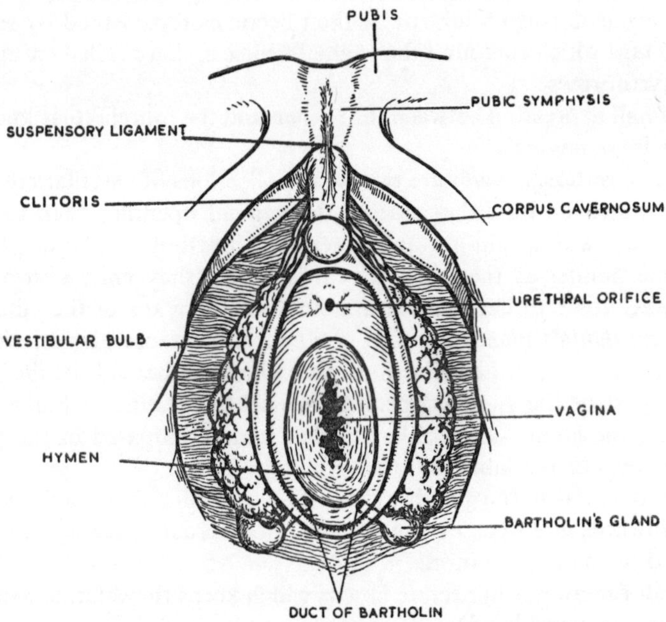

FIGURE 2. Diagram of clitoris and vestibular bulbs

(e) *The vestibule* is the narrow cleft lying between the labia minora, which must be separated to bring it into view. It contains the openings of the urethra above and the vagina below.

(f) *The urethral meatus* is a small opening lying about one inch below the clitoris in the anterior part of the vestibule. In appearance it is a small vertical slit with slightly prominent margins. Two small dimples are usually present on each side of the orifice—these are the openings of Skene's tubules. These structures are two small blind tubules which run for about a quarter of an inch parallel to the course of the urethra within its wall.

(g) *The vaginal orifice* is also known as the introitus vaginae and occupies the lower two-thirds of the vestibule, lying between the labia minora. In the virgin it is covered by an incomplete membrane known as the hymen.

(h) *The hymen* is a membrane, present from birth, which closes the vaginal orifice. Its function is to prevent the entry of urine into the vagina. The central portion is defective so that a hole is present which allows the menstrual discharge to drain away.

The hymen is ruptured at the time of marriage and further lacerations occur during childbirth. It then becomes represented by small fleshy tags which surround the vaginal orifice and are called carunculae myrtiformes.

A small depression between the hymen and the fourchette is known as the fossa navicularis.

(i) *The vestibular bulbs* are two small collections of vascular erectile tissue which lie on either side of the vaginal opening, deep to the labia majora and minora, and anterior to Bartholin's glands. They become thinner as they pass forwards, where they unite above the urethral orifice to become continuous with the glans of the clitoris.

(j) *Bartholin's glands* are two compound racemose glands, about the size and shape of small beans, which lie on either side of the posterior part of the vaginal opening, behind the vestibular bulbs and deep to the labia. When enlarged they can be palpated in the posterior third of the labia majora.

The ducts from the glands are lined by transitional epithelium and pass inwards and open on the surface just external to the hymen and medial to the labia minora.

Their function is to excrete mucus which keeps the external genital organs moist and lubricated.

Both the vestibular bulbs and Bartholin's glands rest upon a deeper structure known as the triangular ligament or the perineal membrane.

The vulva is supplied with blood from two main arteries:

(i) The femoral artery, in the upper part of the thigh. This sends branches known as the superficial and deep external pudendal arteries into the vulva.

(ii) The internal pudendal artery, running along the pubic arch. This terminates in branches which supply the vulva, known as the posterior labial and the deep and dorsal arteries of the clitoris.

The veins drain to corresponding veins.

Lymphatic vessels pass to the horizontal groups of inguinal glands, some passing directly to the external iliac groups.

The skin of the vulva is supplied by the ilio-inguinal nerve, the genital branch of the genito-femoral nerve and the perineal branch of the posterior cutaneous nerve of the thigh. It also receives branches from the posterior labial nerves and the dorsal nerve of the clitoris, which are derived from the pudendal nerve.

THE VAGINA

The vagina is a tube which leads from the vulva to the uterus, passing upwards and backwards into the pelvis, approximately parallel to the plane of the pelvic brim. It is partially closed at its lower end (in virgins) by the hymen. At its upper end it is attached to the cervix of the uterus, which projects almost at a right angle into the upper part of its anterior wall, thus making the posterior wall of the vagina longer (four inches, 10·1 cm.) than the anterior wall (three inches, 7·6 cm). The recesses of the vagina which surround the projecting cervix are named the fornices of the vagina. They are four in number, and are known, according to their positions, as the anterior, posterior and lateral fornices. As the vagina is attached to the cervix at a higher level behind than in front, it makes the posterior fornix larger and more voluminous than either the anterior fornix or the two lateral fornices.

Although the vagina is here described as a tube its lumen is not normally patent, but instead the anterior and posterior walls lie in close contact. They easily become separated to allow the passage of blood during menstruation and the foetus during parturition.

Structure

On inspection the vaginal walls are seen to be pink in colour. Their texture is not smooth as they are composed of numerous transverse small folds or ridges, which are known as rugae. Their function is to enable the vagina to enlarge. This occurs during parturition when they become stretched out and obliterated, thereby allowing the vagina to accommodate the foetus during its passage to the vulva.

The walls are composed of the following structures:

(i) *A layer of squamous epithelium*, which lines the cavity of the vagina.

(ii) *A vascular layer of elastic connective tissue.*

(iii) *A weak inner coat of smooth muscle tissue*, the cells of which run in a circular direction around the vagina.

(iv) *A stronger outer coat of smooth muscle*, whose fibres pass longitudinally along the vagina. These two layers, however, are not clearly demarcated.

(v) *An encircling layer of connective tissue*, containing blood vessels, lymphatics and nerves, which is part of the visceral pelvic fascia.

Contents

There are no glands situated in the walls of the vagina, which cannot therefore be said to have a lining of mucous membrane. The vagina, however, contains a small amount of fluid which is derived from two sources: it comes partly from the glands of the cervix which excrete an alkaline mucus, and partly from the vaginal blood-vessels which allow serous fluid to transude through the vaginal walls into its lumen. Despite the alkalinity of the cervical mucus the vaginal fluid is acid in reaction having a pH of about 4·5 during reproductive life—this is due to the presence of lactic acid, in a concentration of 0·3 per cent. It is produced by bacterial action from glycogen contained in the cells of the squamous epithelium lining the vagina. These organisms are known as Döderlein's bacilli, and are normal inhabitants of the healthy vagina. If they are absent or reduced in number, as occurs in youth and old age, the vagina is less acid, or even alkaline, and infections such as vulvo-vaginitis in young girls and senile vaginitis in elderly women are prone to occur.

This vaginal acidity has a useful function, for any pathogenic organisms which may invade the vagina are largely destroyed, so maintaining the upper part of the genital tract in a healthy state free from harmful bacteria.

Relations

The vagina has important anatomical relations:

1. *Anterior*. The urethra and Skene's tubules are in close relation to the lower half of the vagina, where they lie embedded in the vaginal wall; the base of the bladder lies in front of its upper half. The pelvic peritoneum does not come into direct contact with the anterior wall.

2. *Posterior*. The perineal body forms the immediate relation of the lowest third of the posterior wall, and separates it from the anal canal. The posterior relation of the middle third is the rectum itself, whilst behind the upper third of the posterior wall lies the peritoneum forming the pouch of Douglas.

3. *Lateral*. The upper two-thirds of the vagina are related laterally to the pelvic fascia, embedded in which run blood-vessels, lymphatics and nerves. The two ureters pass close to the lateral fornices on their way to the bladder.

The lateral relations of the lowest third are mainly muscular, consisting of the two levator ani muscles which pass on either side of the vagina, and the bulbo-cavernosus muscles which lie below them, encircling the introitus vaginae. The vestibular bulbs and Bartholin's glands are also lateral relations of the vaginal opening.

4. *Superior*. The upper relation of the vagina is the uterus, the cervix being inserted into the upper part of its anterior wall.

5. *Inferior*. Below the vagina lies the hymen or the carunculae myrtiformes, and the structures of the vulva.

The blood-supply to the vagina comes from the vaginal, the uterine (descending branch), the middle haemorrhoidal, the inferior vesical and pudendal arteries—all branches of the internal iliac artery. The veins drain in a corresponding manner.

The lymphatics of the lowest third drain to the horizontal inguinal groups along with those of the vulva; from the upper two-thirds they pass to the internal iliac and sacral glands.

The nerve supply is formed by the sympathetic and para-sympathetic systems from the plexus of Lee-Frankenhäuser.

THE UTERUS

The uterus is a hollow, flattened, muscular, pear-shaped organ which lies in the true pelvis above the vagina, receiving the insertions of the two Fallopian tubes into its upper and outer angles. It measures 3 inches (7·6 cm.) in length, 2 inches (5·1 cm.) in width at its widest part and 1 inch (2·5 cm.) in depth, whilst its walls are ½ inch (1·3 cm.) in thickness. The uterine cavity is therefore 2½ inches (6·4 cm.) long. The uterus weighs about two ounces (56 g.). It consists of the following parts:

(a) *The body or corpus*, which comprises the upper two-thirds of the uterus. The cavity of the body is triangular in shape with its base directed upwards. Owing to the flattening of the uterus, its anterior and posterior walls are normally in contact.

(b) *The neck or cervix*, which forms the lowest third of the uterus and is therefore one inch (2·5 cm.) in length. The cavity here is narrow and slightly fusiform in shape, being known as the cervical canal. Its widest part lies in the centre of the cervix, and it is more constricted above where it is continuous with the cavity of the body through the

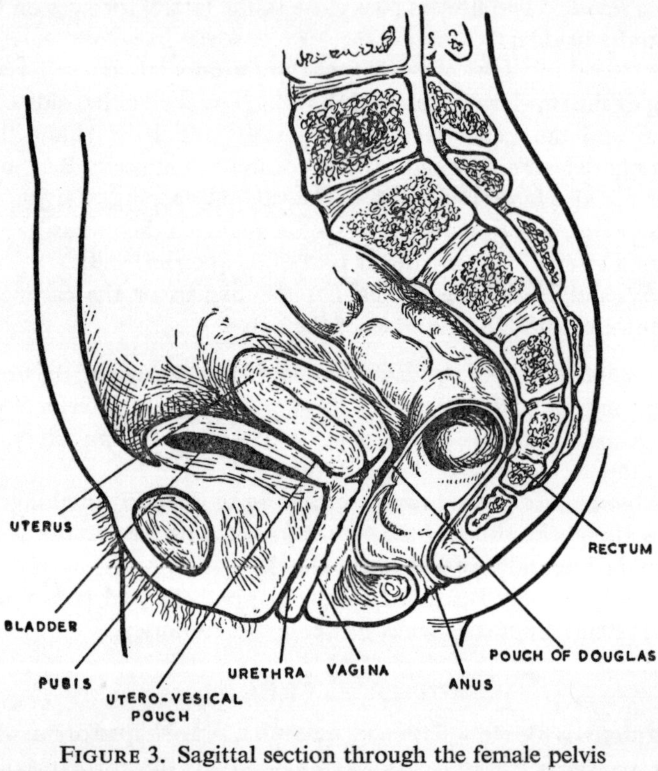

FIGURE 3. Sagittal section through the female pelvis

internal os, and below where it communicates with the vagina through the external os.

(c) *The isthmus*, which is a narrow zone of the corpus uteri, about seven mm. in length, situated in its lowest part immediately above the internal os. It has a special function during pregnancy, which is described in Chapter 8.

(d) *The fundus*, which is the portion of the body of the uterus lying between the insertions of the two Fallopian tubes.

(e) *The cornua*, which is the name applied to the lateral angles of the uterine body where the Fallopian tubes are attached.

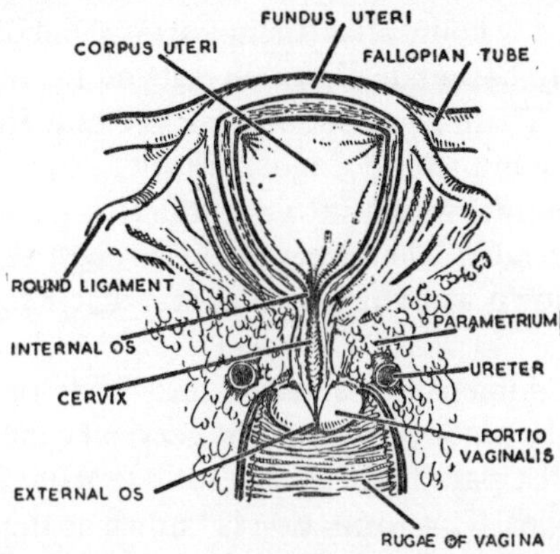

FIGURE 4. Dissection to show the opened cavity of the body of the uterus, the cervical canal and the upper part of the vagina. Note the position of the ureters lateral to the cervix

Structure

The uterus is a muscular organ, and its walls are chiefly composed of plain muscle cells. This part of the uterus is known as the myometrium. The uterine cavity is lined by mucous membrane which is called the endometrium, whilst the peritoneum which covers the body of the uterus may be referred to as the perimetrium.

A. THE ENDOMETRIUM

This is the mucous membrane which lines the interior of the uterus. The mucosa of the uterine body differs markedly from that of the cervical canal, their chief features being as follows:

(a) *The corporeal endometrium* consists of a vascular connective tissue, known as the stroma, in which are contained numerous mucus-secreting tubular glands which open into the uterine cavity. The stroma is covered by a layer of cubical cells which form the glands by dipping down in finger-like processes into the stroma. On the surface these cells are ciliated. The endometrium varies in thickness and vascularity from day to day according to the phases of the menstrual cycle, and it is largely shed during the actual process of menstruation. This is described in Chapter 4. The endometrium of the isthmus is thinner than that of the rest of the corpus, and as it has fewer glands and blood-vessels, is of generally poorer quality.

(b) *The cervical endometrium* is much thinner than that of the body and is made up of a connective tissue stroma lined by tall ciliated columnar cells with basal nuclei, which rests on the muscle and collagen of the cervix. There is no submucosa present. In places the epithelium forms deep branching glands, known as compound racemose glands, which penetrate deeply into the underlying tissue. They sometimes become distended when they bulge through the surface of the cervix and are known as ovules of Naboth. Their function is to excrete mucus.

The cervical endometrium is raised into folds or ridges: one of these runs down the anterior wall of the cervical canal and one down the posterior, whilst parallel branches radiate from both in upward and lateral directions. This formation is known as the arbor vitae and it is believed to facilitate the passage of spermatozoa from the vagina to the body of the uterus. This membrane does not change markedly during the menstrual cycle.

B. The Myometrium

This constitutes the main mass of the uterus, and in the body is made up of plain muscle cells which run in bundles separated by connective tissue. The muscle bundles pass in all directions in an interlacing manner (when the patient is not pregnant), and surround the blood-vessels and lymphatics passing to and from the endometrium. The outermost muscle fibres become continuous with those of the uterine ligaments and the longitudinal fibres of the Fallopian tubes and vagina.

In the cervix, however, the muscle bundles are less numerous and compact, and they lie embedded in a groundwork of collagen fibres. Some muscle fibres form a continuous band running from the body of the uterus to the vagina, which constitutes the 'extrinsic' muscle of the cervix; other more immature fibres radiate towards the mucosa and the lips of the cervix, and comprise the 'intrinsic' muscle.

C. The Perimetrium

This is the outer covering of the uterus which consists of peritoneum. A full description of the distribution of the pelvic peritoneum is given later.

Attachments

(i) The vagina is related to the uterus below, where the cervix pro-

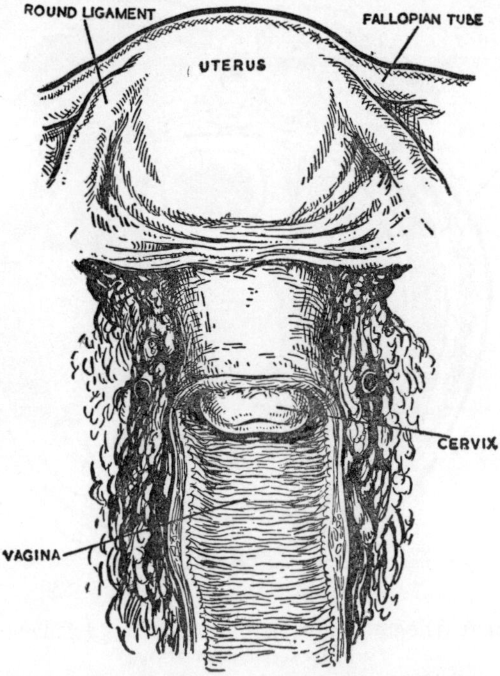

FIGURE 5. Anterior view of uterus and vagina, showing the cervix and vaginal fornices

jects into its upper part and so creates the vaginal fornices. The vaginal wall is attached half-way along the length of the cervix, so that it becomes divided into two approximately equal halves, the supra-vaginal cervix situated above the vagina, and the vaginal cervix lying within its lumen. The vaginal portion of the cervix, known as the portio vaginalis, is covered by squamous epithelium similar to that which lines the vagina itself; this becomes continuous with the columnar epithelium of the cervical canal at the external os.

(ii) At the upper part of the uterus the Fallopian tubes are attached to the uterus in the regions of the cornua.

(iii) As is explained in Chapter 2, the upper two-thirds of the vagina and the cervix are surrounded by visceral pelvic fascia, which may be thought of as packing material, filling the spaces between the various pelvic organs. In places this fascia becomes condensed into strong bands which run from the uterus and the vagina to the pelvic walls. These bands contain smooth muscle fibres which have contractile

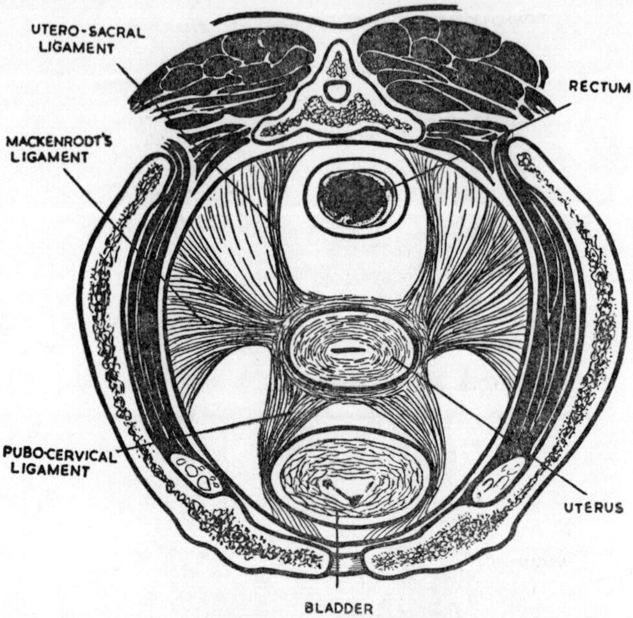

FIGURE 6. Diagram showing the supporting ligaments of the uterus seen from above

and supporting functions; they are known as uterine ligaments and help to maintain this organ in its normal position.

The Uterine Ligaments

(a) *The two cardinal ligaments,* also known as the transverse cervical ligaments and Mackenrodt's ligaments, run in a radiating fan-like manner from the lateral aspect of the cervix below the level of the internal os and the lateral fornices of the vagina to the side walls of the pelvis, where they are attached to the fascia overlying the obturator internus muscles. The ureters on their way to the bladder pass through these ligaments, lying in what are known as the ureteric canals.

(b) *The two utero-sacral ligaments* pass from the cervix in an upward and backward direction, and encircle the rectum to become attached to the periosteum of the sacrum.

(c) *The two pubo-cervical ligaments* are a pair of weak ligaments which run forwards from the cervix, underneath the bladder, to become attached to the pubic bones. Some authorities deny that they exist.

(d) *The two round ligaments* begin at the cornua of the uterus, pass downwards, forwards and outwards within the broad ligaments, and then cross the lateral parts of the pelvic floor to reach the internal inguinal rings, situated above the inguinal ligaments in the anterior abdominal wall. They then turn medially around the deep epigastric vessels and enter the inguinal canals in the groins. They traverse the canals, emerge through the external rings in the oblique muscles, and end in the fatty tissues of the labia majora.

These ligaments are of embryological interest, for they mark the route along which the testes descend in the male, in whom the scrotum corresponds to the fused labia majora.

(e) *The two ovarian ligaments* also begin at the cornua of the uterus and pass downwards, backwards and outwards inside the broad ligaments for about an inch to become connected to the ovaries. They help to suspend the ovaries in their normal position and keep them steady whilst ovulation is occurring.

The ovarian and round ligaments form one continuous ligament during early foetal life, and are derived from a common origin, known as the gubernaculum ovarii.

(f) *The two broad ligaments.* Although these are mentioned here for the sake of completeness, it must be clearly understood that they are not condensations of pelvic fascia, but are, instead, folds of peritoneum passing laterally from the uterus to the side walls of the pelvis. They are not true ligaments in any way, and are more fully described later.

The uterus and pelvic cellular tissue lie in the pelvis above the levator ani muscles (described in Chapter 2), which form a platform to support them in their normal positions. When these muscles relax, as during defaecation, the ligaments act as direct supports of the uterus, the most important in this way being the cardinal ligaments.

Position

The uterus is situated in the true pelvis between the bladder in front and below, and the pouch of Douglas and rectum behind. The cervix lies approximately on an imaginary line joining the ischial spines. In 80 per cent of individuals the uterus inclines forwards over

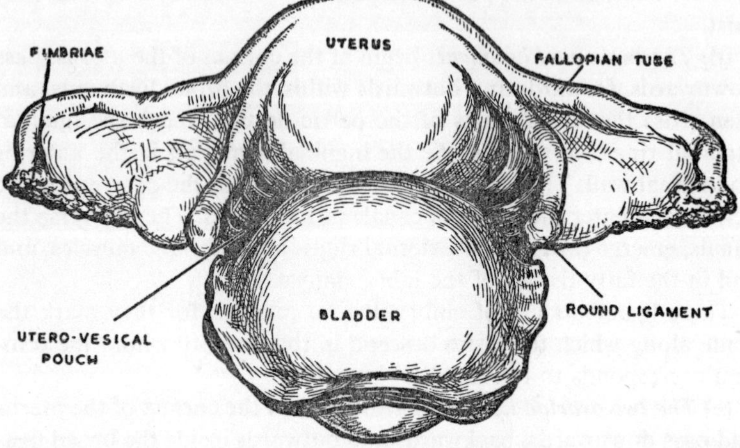

FIGURE 7. Anterior view of uterus and bladder, showing the peritoneal relationships

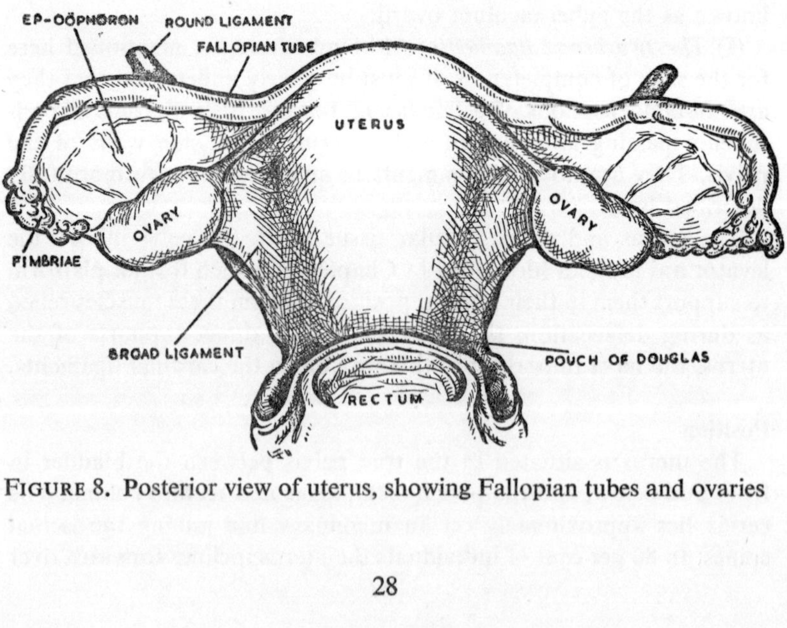

FIGURE 8. Posterior view of uterus, showing Fallopian tubes and ovaries

the upper surface of the bladder, and is said to lie in a position of anteversion.

The maintenance of this position is helped by the supporting action of the utero-sacral ligaments behind and the round ligaments in front. In 20 per cent of individuals the reverse position is present and the uterus then inclines backwards, this being known as retroversion.

In addition to this inclination, the body of the uterus may bend forwards or backwards on the cervix at the level of the internal os. This is known as anteflexion or retroflexion of the uterus respectively —the former is the commoner.

Relations

(a) *Anterior*. The bladder is placed anterior to the cervix with the pubo-cervical ligaments below it. The utero-vesical pouch of peritoneum and coils of intestine lie in front of the body, above the bladder.

(b) *Posterior*. The posterior surface of the uterus is in relation to the peritoneal cavity, the portion lying below the utero-sacral folds of peritoneum being known as the pouch of Douglas. The utero-sacral ligaments are also posterior relations.

(c) *Lateral*. Lateral to the body of the uterus are the broad ligaments, the Fallopian tubes, ovaries and round ligaments.

Lateral to the cervix, running in the pelvic fascia, lie the ureters which are passing forwards to the bladder; alongside the cervix they are crossed above by the uterine vessels which are passing from the side walls of the pelvis to supply the uterus.

(d) *Superior*. The intestines.

(e) *Inferior*. The vagina. The fornices can be said to form the immediate relations of the vaginal cervix.

The blood supply of the body of the uterus comes from the uterine and ovarian arteries and returns via corresponding veins. The cervix is supplied by descending branches from the uterine arteries and is drained by the uterine veins.

The lymph drainage of the body is into the internal iliac glands, with small vessels passing along the round ligaments to the horizontal inguinal glands. Lymph from the cervix drains first into the parametrial glands, lying alongside the cervix in the visceral pelvic fascia, and then to the internal iliac and sacral glands. A few lymphatic vessels pass first to the obturator glands lying in the obturator fossa in the upper part of the foramen ovale and then to the internal iliac glands.

The nerve supply is through the Lee-Frankenhäuser plexus, being derived from the sympathetic and para-sympathetic systems. A few ganglia lie alongside the cervix.

THE FALLOPIAN TUBES

These are two small tubes, each about four inches (10·1 cm.) long and one-quarter of an inch (6 mm.) in diameter, which are attached to the cornua of the uterus. They pass laterally from the uterus across the pelvis almost to reach its side walls, where they turn backwards and downwards towards the ovaries. The tubes possess a lumen which communicates with the cavity of the uterus medially and which opens into the peritoneal cavity laterally. The female genital tract is thus an open pathway which leads from the exterior to the peritoneal cavity via the vulva, vagina, uterus and Fallopian tubes.

The tubes can be considered to consist of four parts:

1. *The interstitial part*, which is the narrowest part of the tube, having a lumen of one mm., lying within the thickness of the uterine wall.

2. *The isthmus*, which also is a narrow portion of the tube extending for about one inch (2·5 cm.) laterally from the uterine wall.

3. *The ampulla*, which is much wider than the isthmus and extends for about two inches (5·1 cm.) laterally from the isthmus towards the side wall of the pelvis.

4. *The infundibulum*, which is the lateral inch (2·5 cm.) of the tube which turns backwards and downwards. It is composed of numerous finger-like processes, the fimbriae, which surround the tubal orifice. One fimbria is attached to the ovary and is known as the fimbria ovarica. A small pedunculated vesicular structure is sometimes attached to the fimbriated extremity of the tube—this is named the hydatid of Morgagni.

Attachments

The tubes are attached medially to the uterus, and as they pass transversely across the pelvis they carry with them the peritoneum. This is draped across them forming a fold which passes down to the pelvic floor below, so constituting the broad ligaments.

Where the lateral extremities of the tubes bend backwards, the peritoneum is continued as folds to the side walls of the pelvis, producing what are known as the infundibulo-pelvic ligaments. It can thus be appreciated that these are peritoneal structures and not true ligaments, although they do accord some means of support both to the Fallopian tubes and ovaries. They also transmit the ovarian vessels, lymphatics and nerves.

Structure

The Fallopian tube is a true tube although this would hardly be

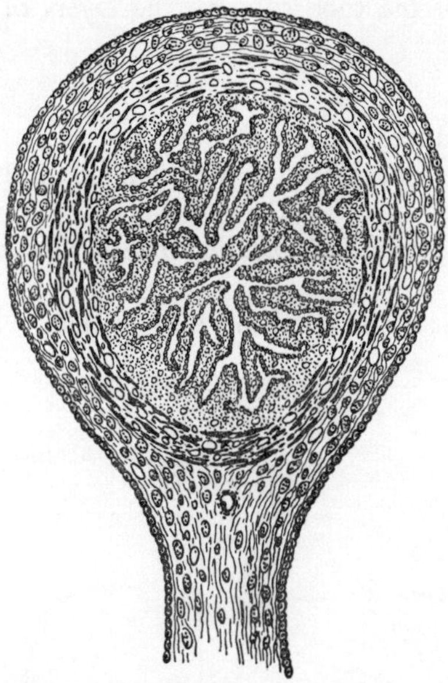

FIGURE 9. Cross-section of Fallopian tube

suspected from looking at its cross-section under the microscope, because its mucous membrane is thrown into such rich and profuse folds that its lumen is not obvious. These folds, which are known as plicae, are most developed in the ampullary portions of the tubes, where they act as a device which serves to slow down the passage of the ovum during its journey to the uterus.

The parts of the tube outside the uterus are made up of the following layers:

(i) A layer of cubical epithelium, many cells of which are ciliated, which covers the plicae throughout all their intricacies. Some of the non-ciliated cells are known as goblet cells and contain large globules of secretion; these are discharged into the lumen of the tube shortly before menstruation, after which the cells collapse and are then called peg cells.

(ii) A vascular layer of connective tissue, which lies below the surface epithelium.

(iii) An inner layer of circular smooth muscle which surrounds the mucous membrane.

(iv) An outer layer of longitudinal smooth muscle.

(v) An outer covering of peritoneum, which is absent along the inferior surface of the tube between the layers of the broad ligament.

Relations

(i) *Medial.* The uterus.

(ii) *Lateral.* The infundibulo-pelvic ligaments and the side walls of the pelvis.

(iii) *Anterior, superior and posterior.* The peritoneal cavity and the intestines.

(iv) *Inferior.* The broad ligaments and ovaries.

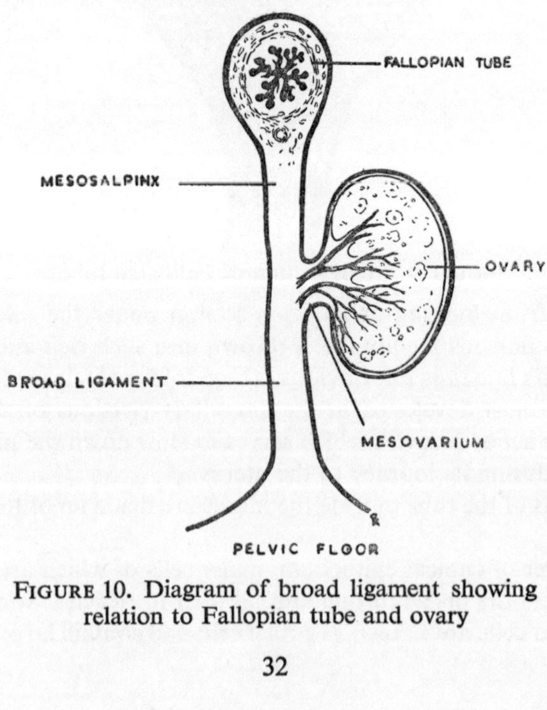

FIGURE 10. Diagram of broad ligament showing relation to Fallopian tube and ovary

The tubes are supplied with blood from the uterine and ovarian arteries, and drain via corresponding veins.

The lymphatics pass with those of the ovary to the lumbar glands.

The nerve supply is mainly from the ovarian plexus.

THE OVARIES

The ovary is an organ whose structure and function vary at different ages of the individual. These changes are described in Chapter 4, and the anatomical description now given is that of the ovary during the child-bearing period of life.

The ovaries are two small almond-shaped bodies, dull white in colour and corrugated on the surface, measuring 3 cm. in length, 2 cm. in breadth and 1 cm. in thickness and weighing about 6 grammes. They are attached to the posterior layer of the broad ligaments, and lie inside the peritoneal cavity. They sometimes rest in a small depression in the parietal peritoneum on the lateral wall of the pelvis below the bifurcation of the common iliac artery, which is known as the ovarian fossa of Waldeyer. The lateral portion of the Fallopian tube arches over the ovary and ends in close proximity to it, being connected to it by the fimbria ovarica. When the uterus is retroverted the ovaries may lie in the pouch of Douglas.

Attachments

The place of attachment of the ovary to the posterior layer of the broad ligament is known as the mesovarium, and the part of the broad ligament extending above this point to the Fallopian tube is called the mesosalpinx.

This attachment however is too weak to support the ovary, which is suspended from the uterine cornu by the ovarian ligament. As described above this is a strong structure, containing smooth muscle, which runs inside the broad ligament to be attached to the ovary through the medial margin of the mesovarium.

Similarly the lateral pole of the ovary is supported by the infundibulo-pelvic ligament, which has already been described as a fold of peritoneum running to the side wall of the pelvis and transmitting the ovarian vessels, lymphatics and nerves.

Structure

The ovary consists of a medulla and cortex surrounded by a layer of germinal epithelium.

(i) *The medulla* is the part of the ovary which is directly attached to the broad ligament at the mesovarium. It consists of fibrous tissue and transmits the ovarian vessels, lymphatics and nerves which enter and leave the ovary from the broad ligament, which they have reached through the infundibulo-pelvic ligament.

(ii) *The cortex* is the functional part of the ovary and consists of a dense stroma in which are situated ovarian follicles and corpora lutea in various stages of development and retrogression. These structures are more fully described in Chapter 4. The outer part of the cortex is formed by a dense fibrous coat, which is known as the tunica albuginea.

(iii) *The germinal epithelium* consists of a layer of low cubical cells which covers the tunica albuginea of the cortex, and is continuous with the peritoneum of the broad ligament at the mesovarium. It may be said to be a modified form of the peritoneum which covers the ovary.

Relations

(i) *Medial.* The body of the uterus and the ovarian ligament running to the cornu.

(ii) *Lateral.* The infundibulo-pelvic ligament and the side wall of the pelvis, covered by parietal peritoneum. The ureter and internal iliac artery form the posterior boundary of the fossa of Waldeyer in which the ovary rests whilst the obliterated hypogastric artery forms its anterior margin.

(iii) *Anterior.* The broad ligament and the mesovarium.

(iv) *Posterior.* The peritoneal cavity and the intestines.

The blood-supply is from the ovarian arteries. The ovarian veins join the inferior vena cava on the right and the left renal vein on the left.

The lymph drainage is into the lumbar glands.

The nerve supply is from the ovarian plexus.

THE PELVIC PERITONEUM

The anatomy of the female internal genital organs cannot be properly understood unless their relation to the distribution of the pelvic peritoneum is clearly borne in mind. This is somewhat complex in the female and is best learnt by comparison with its distribution in the more simple male pelvis.

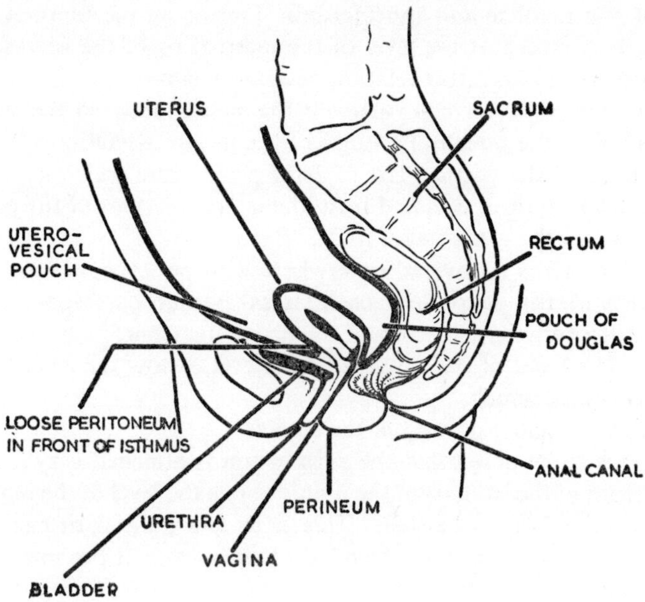

FIGURE 11. Diagram showing distribution of Pelvic Peritoneum

In males, the peritoneum lines the anterior abdominal wall, extends down on to the upper surface of the bladder and then passes on to the rectum and the posterior abdominal wall. In the female pelvis the uterus, tubes and ovaries are placed transversely across the pelvis between the bladder and rectum; consequently the peritoneum first passes on to the upper surface of the bladder, then passes up the anterior surface of the uterus, over the fundus and down the posterior surface as far as the junction of the upper and middle thirds of the posterior wall of the vagina. It then passes on to the rectum and posterior abdominal wall as in the male. The uterus, however, only occupies the median plane of the pelvis and the Fallopian tubes spread out on either side of it as far as the lateral pelvic walls. Consequently, lateral to the uterus, the peritoneum rises up to the Fallopian tubes, arches over their upper border and then descends behind them, so forming the broad ligaments. The uterus and broad ligaments thus form a partition across the pelvis which divides it into anterior and posterior compartments. Certain details of this arrangement are to be specially noted:

(i) In the anterior compartment the pouch between the upper surface of the bladder and the uterus is known as the utero-vesical pouch. It is placed at the level of the internal os of the uterus and does not come into direct relation with the vagina.

(ii) In the posterior compartment the pouch between the uterus and rectum is the pouch of Douglas. It is in direct relation with the upper third of the vagina. The folds of peritoneum which lie above the utero-sacral ligaments and form the lateral margins of the pouch are known as the utero-sacral folds.

(iii) The uterus is covered everywhere with peritoneum except:

(a) A narrow strip along each lateral border, corresponding to the space between the layers of the broad ligament.

(b) The front of the supravaginal cervix, below the level of the utero-vesical pouch.

(c) The vaginal portion of the cervix.

(iv) It is to be noted that the peritoneum is attached very loosely to the front of the isthmus of the uterus above the level of the internal os, but quite firmly elsewhere. This is to allow the peritoneum to accommodate itself to the distended bladder when it becomes filled with urine.

(v) The peritoneum covers the upper two-thirds of the rectum, lining its anterior aspect in the middle third, and its anterior and lateral aspects in the upper third. The lowest third lies posterior to the middle third of the vagina and is not related to the peritoneum.

The Contents of the Broad Ligament

The space between the two peritoneal layers forming the broad ligament is filled with visceral pelvic fascia and fat, containing the uterine and ovarian vessels and their branches, lymphatics and nerves. In addition other important structures are present:

(i) The Fallopian tube in its upper border.

(ii) The ovarian ligament.

(iii) The round ligament.

(iv) The ureter. This passes forwards through the base of the broad ligament lateral to the cervix, close to the lateral fornix of the vagina. In this position it passes through Mackenrodt's ligament in a special tunnel, known as the ureteric canal.

(v) The epoöphoron, paroöphoron and Gärtner's duct comprising the organ of Rosenmüller. These are embryonic structures, corresponding to the ducts of the male reproductive system, which persist in a rudimentary fashion in the female. They are present in the mesosalpinx, and Gärtner's duct, when well formed, runs down the lateral border of the uterus into the lateral wall of the vagina.

Vestigial Structures in the Broad Ligament

During the process of development of the human body three separate sets of kidneys are formed. The first two which appear in early embryonic life form the pronephros; after a while these atrophy and are replaced by the second pair known as the mesonephros. These in their turn atrophy and are replaced by the third pair, the metanephros, which persist and function throughout life.

These early kidneys may leave remnants behind which are functionless and are known as vestigial structures. Thus the hydatid of Morgagni, and a few tubules occurring close to it known as Kobelt's tubules, are remains of the pronephros, whilst the organ of Rosenmüller mentioned above is all that is left of the mesonephros, the duct of Gärtner being the mesonephric ureter.

In the male the mesonephros and its duct form the epididymis and the vas deferens, which are used to conduct spermatozoa from the testis to the urethra.

CHAPTER 2

The Anatomy and Physiology of other Pelvic Contents

THE URETERS

The ureters are two narrow tubes, about 10 in. (25·4 cm.) in length and $\frac{1}{8}$ in. (3 mm.) in diameter, that convey the urine from the pelves of the kidneys to the bladder. They are essentially muscular in nature, and waves of peristalsis pass along them propelling the urine into the bladder, in much the same way that the gut contents are driven forwards by intestinal peristalsis.

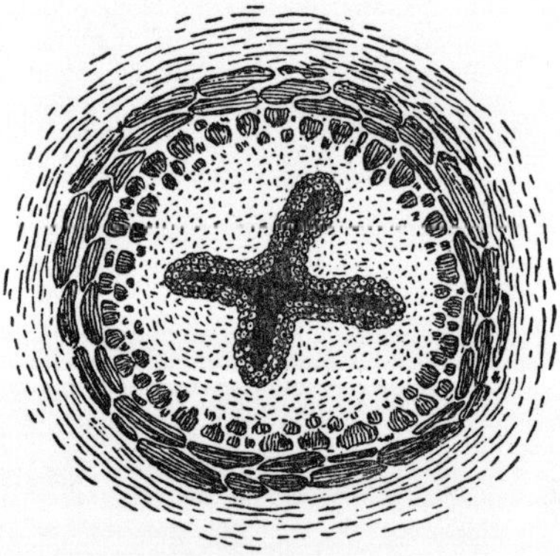

FIGURE 12. Section of ureter

Structure

The wall of the ureter as it passes through the pelvis is composed of the following layers:

(i) A coat of transitional epithelium which lines the lumen of the tube and forms longitudinal folds.

(ii) A fibrous tissue layer containing many elastic fibres, on which the epithelium rests.

(iii) An inner weak layer of longitudinal smooth muscle fibres.

(iv) A middle circular layer of smooth muscle.

(v) A well-defined outer layer of longitudinal muscle.

(vi) A coat of fibrous connective tissue.

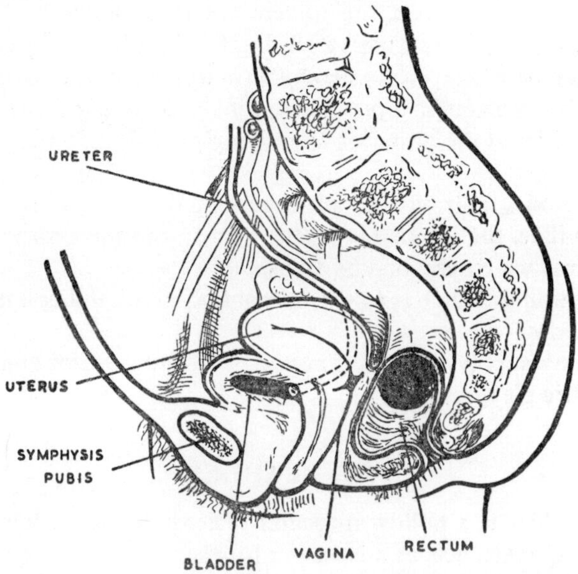

FIGURE 13. Side wall of pelvis, showing course of ureter

Course

Throughout their whole course the ureters are placed outside the peritoneum.

They begin at the kidneys and pass down in the posterior abdominal wall towards the pelvis. They cross the pelvic brim anterior to the sacro-iliac joint and enter the true pelvis by passing over the common iliac arteries at the point where these divide into the external and internal iliac arteries. The ureters then pass down the side walls of the pelvis lying in front of the internal iliac arteries, and forming the posterior margin of the ovarian fossae. In this part of their course they lie internal to the superior vesical vessels, the obturator nerve, artery and vein, and the inferior vesical vessels.

The ureters then turn medially and forwards at the level of the ischial spines and run through the pelvic fascia above the upper surface of the levator ani muscles to the bladder. In this region they pass through the bases of the broad ligaments, special tunnels (the ureteric canals) running through Mackenrodt's ligaments. Here they lie lateral to the cervix and close to the lateral fornices of the vagina, and the uterine vessels, on their way from the side walls of the pelvis, cross over them.

In front of the cervix the ureters enter the bladder. They run obliquely for about $\frac{3}{4}$ in. (19 mm.) through the bladder wall, this device serving as a mechanism whereby urinary regurgitation from the bladder into the ureters is prevented. Finally they open into the cavity of the bladder at the posterior lateral angles of the trigone.

The blood supply in the pelvic part of their course is from the common iliac, the internal iliac, the uterine and the vesical arteries, and returns via corresponding veins.

The lymph drainage is to the internal, external and common iliac lymph nodes.

The nerve supply is from the aortic, renal and superior and inferior hypogastric plexuses.

THE BLADDER

The bladder is a hollow muscular distensible organ, lying in the true pelvis, which acts as a reservoir for the storage of urine prior to micturition. It is roughly pyramidal in shape when empty, having a base or trigone which rests on the vagina, and an upper surface, continuous with the floor of the utero-vesical pouch, which extends from the cervix to the upper border of the symphysis pubis. The anterior part of the upper surface is sometimes termed the apex of the bladder. It has two infero-lateral surfaces which rest on the upper surface of the levator ani muscles.

The trigone of the bladder is triangular in shape, with its base placed behind and its apex in front. Each of its three sides measures about one inch (2·5 cm.) in length. At the extremities of the base are placed the ureteric orifices—these are narrow slit-like apertures, through which the ureters open after having obliquely penetrated the bladder wall. The apex of the trigone is formed by the internal meatus where the urethra leaves the bladder. This region is known as the bladder neck.

The normal capacity of the bladder is twenty ounces (568 ml.), though under pathological conditions it may contain many litres of urine when its shape becomes more globular, and its upper part rises into the abdomen.

Structure

The bladder walls are formed by the following layers:

1. The cavity is lined by transitional epithelium which rests on a layer of areolar tissue. The epithelium is thrown into folds or rugae, similar to those of the vaginal walls, to allow for distension; this arrangement however is absent over the trigone, where the epithelium is firmly bound down to the subjacent muscle.

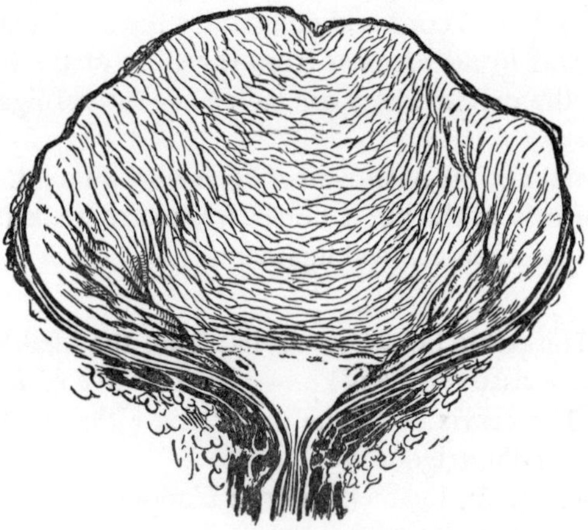

FIGURE 14. Dissection of the bladder showing the trigone, the ureteric orifices and the internal meatus

2. The epithelium of the bladder is surrounded by three coats of smooth muscle, which are arranged as inner longitudinal, middle circular and outer longitudinal layers. This muscle is known as the detrusor muscle, and is so called because when it contracts it expels the urine from the bladder during the act of micturition. The circular muscle is thickened around the internal meatus to form the internal sphincter of the bladder. It is in a constant state of contraction except during micturition.

The muscles in the trigone of the bladder have a rather especial arrangement. The muscle fibres running between the ureteric orifices are collected into a band which is known as the interureteric (Mercier's) bar. The muscle fibres passing from the ureteric orifices to the internal meatus are called the muscles of Bell; they pass into the urethra through the internal meatus and play an important role during the act of micturition.

3. The upper surface of the bladder is covered with peritoneum, whilst its remaining surfaces are invested with visceral pelvic fascia.

The Ligaments of the Bladder

Five ligaments are attached to the bladder:

1. *A fibrous band* known as the urachus runs from the apex of the bladder up the anterior abdominal wall to the umbilicus. During foetal life this structure is patent, when it passes through the umbilicus into the umbilical cord and constitutes the allantois.

2. *Two fibrous ligaments* pass from the sides of the bladder to the side walls of the pelvis. These are called the lateral ligaments of the bladder.

3. *Two ligaments, the pubo-vesical ligaments,* attach the neck of the bladder anteriorly to the pubic bones. These are weak structures and form part of the pubo-cervical ligaments.

Relations

Anterior. The pubic bones, separated from the bladder by a space filled with fatty tissue—this is known as the Cave of Retzius.

Posterior. The cervix, with the ureters on either side entering the lateral angles of the trigone.

Lateral. The lateral ligaments of the bladder and the side walls of the pelvis.

Superior. The body of the anteverted uterus and the intestines lying in the utero-vesical pouch.

Inferior. The upper half of the anterior vaginal wall lying below the trigone, and the levator ani muscles situated below the infero-lateral surfaces.

The blood-supply is from the superior and inferior vesical arteries, with a few twigs from the uterine and vaginal arteries. The veins drain into corresponding vessels.

The lymph drainage is into the external iliac glands and obturator glands.

The nerve supply is from the sympathetic and para-sympathetic systems, through the Lee-Frankenhäuser plexus.

THE URETHRA

The urethra is a narrow tube, one and a half inches (3·8 cm.) in length, which passes from the internal meatus of the bladder to open into the vestibule.

Course

It runs practically embedded in the lower half of the anterior vaginal wall. At its origin from the bladder it is surrounded by a thickening of the circular muscle of the bladder which functions as an internal sphincter. It then passes between the two levator ani muscles, and below these it is enclosed by bands of striated muscle, known as the membranous sphincter of the urethra, which although it is not a true external sphincter, functions in that capacity.

Structure

The wall of the urethra contains the following layers:

1. The lumen is lined by transitional epithelium in its upper half and squamous epithelium in its lower half.
2. These epithelia rest on a layer of vascular connective tissue.
3. An inner longitudinal coat of smooth muscle. These muscle fibres are continuous with the inner longitudinal fibres of the bladder, which pass through the internal meatus.
4. An outer circular coat of smooth muscle fibres.

The lumen of the urethra is normally closed, when its wall is thrown into small longitudinal folds. Several minute diverticula or crypts open into the urethra. These run longitudinally in the urethral wall for a short distance and communicate with the lumen of the urethra at their lowest point. The two largest of these are Skene's tubules which open on to the surface just lateral to the urethral orifice in the vestibule. They correspond to the prostate gland in the male.

The blood-supply is from the inferior vesical and pudendal arteries. The veins drain similarly.

The lymph drainage is into the internal iliac glands.

The internal sphincter is supplied by the sympathetic, whilst the membranous sphincter is under voluntary control via the pudendal nerve.

The Physiology of Micturition

When the bladder is filled with about thirteen ounces (300 ml.) of urine, sensations are conveyed to the hypothalamus and cortical centres of the brain through sensory sympathetic nerves, informing the patient that the performance of micturition is necessary. This act can be voluntarily postponed until a suitable moment, although contractions occur in the bladder wall which render the desire for micturition practically irresistible when the volume of urine reaches twenty-five ounces (700 ml.).

When the act is performed the contraction of the internal sphincter by the sympathetic nerves is relaxed, whilst the voluntary nerves relax the membranous sphincter. At the same time the detrusor muscle contracts through stimulation by para-sympathetic nerves, the internal meatus is pulled open by Bell's muscles, the intra-abdominal pressure is increased and the bladder becomes emptied.

THE RECTUM

The rectum is the continuation of the pelvic colon. It begins at the level of the third sacral vertebra, lies in the hollow of the sacrum and ends below at the tip of the coccyx, where it makes a right-angled bend backwards to join the anal canal. It is a distensible tube about five inches (12·7 cm.) in length and wider in its lower part where it forms the rectal ampulla. As it passes downwards it has three bends, two to the right and one to the left, which help to support the weight of the contained faeces. At these bends the mucous membrane forms prominent ridges which are sometimes called the valves of Houston. The rectum is attached to the pelvic wall by condensations of visceral pelvic fascia which form its lateral supporting ligaments.

Structure

The rectal wall consists of the following coats:

1. The cavity is lined by columnar cells which dip down in places into the submucosa to form tubular glands.
2. A vascular submucous layer which lies below the surface epithelium.
3. An inner circular layer of smooth muscle.
4. An outer longitudinal layer of smooth muscle.
5. A peritoneal investment which differs at varying levels:

   (a) The upper third is covered by peritoneum in front and at the sides.

(b) The middle third has a peritoneal lining only in front.

This peritoneal covering of the rectum forms the posterior wall of the pouch of Douglas.

(c) The lowest third has no peritoneal coat.

6. In the places where the peritoneum is absent the rectum is invested with a layer of visceral pelvic fascia.

Relations

Anterior. The pouch of Douglas lies in front of the rectum above, whilst its lowest third is in direct relation with the middle third of the vagina.

Posterior. The sacrum and coccyx.

Lateral. The intestines in the pouch of Douglas. The lateral ligaments of the rectum pass from the lateral borders of the rectum to the pelvic walls, whilst the utero-sacral ligaments encircle the rectum as they pass from the uterus to the sacrum.

The blood supply is from the superior haemorrhoidal (the terminal branch of the inferior mesenteric artery) and the middle haemorrhoidal arteries (from the internal iliac arteries). The veins drain similarly.

The lymph drainage from the lower part of the rectum is into the sacral, the internal iliac and common iliac groups of glands. The upper part drains through vessels which accompany the superior haemorrhoidal vessels to the lymphatic glands lying in the pelvic mesocolon.

The nerve supply is formed by the sympathetic and para-sympathetic systems similar to other pelvic organs.

THE ANAL CANAL

The anal canal is a short tube, about one inch (2·5 cm.) in length, passing from the point where the rectum makes a right-angled turn backwards opposite the tip of the coccyx to end in the anus. During its short course it passes between the levator ani muscles, which in fact encircle it and hold it with a sling-like action in its normal position.

Structure

Although the anal canal is so short, it has a different structure in its upper and lower parts:

1. In its upper two-thirds the anal canal is lined by mucous membrane similar to that of the rectum. This mucosa is not a flat surface but is raised into about six longitudinal folds—the columns of Morgagni. These columns contain veins, which if they become enlarged,

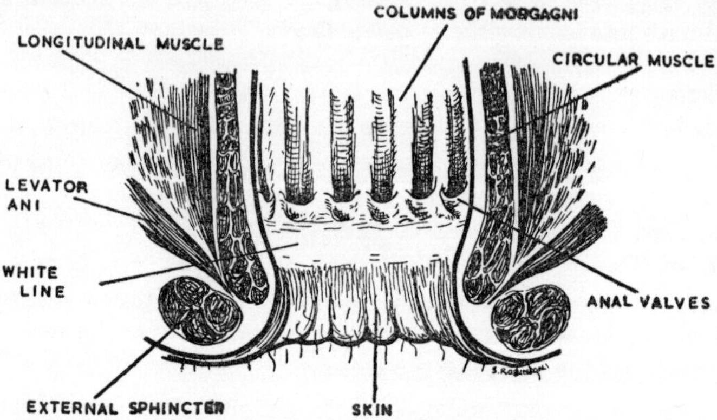

FIGURE 15. Diagram to show the structure of the anal canal

may give rise to internal haemorrhoids. Sometimes these become so large that they prolapse through the anal orifice and become visible on inspection, a frequent occurrence during pregnancy and labour. The lowest ends of the columns are connected by small folds of mucosa which form the anal valves.

2. The lowest third of the anal canal is lined by squamous epithelium continuous with that of the normal skin. Its junction with the mucous membrane above is marked by a distinct white line, called Hilton's line.

3. The muscle coat of the anal canal is arranged in a special manner:

(a) The circular muscle of the rectum is prolonged downwards to surround the anal canal where it becomes thickened to form the internal sphincter of the anus.

(b) A second sphincter is formed by the external sphincter of the anus. This is a striated muscle, partly attached to the coccyx, which surrounds the anus and enters into the formation of the perineal body, thus belonging to the superficial perineal group of muscles.

(c) The longitudinal muscle coat of the rectum joins with the levator ani muscles, which become attached to the anal wall between the two sphincters, where they form a supporting sling.

4. Sometimes small veins external to the anus become dilated and form external piles.

Relations

Superior. The rectum.

Anterior. The perineal body and the lowest third of the vagina.

Posterior. A mass of fibrous tissue lying between the anal canal and the coccyx, known as the ano-coccygeal body.

Lateral. The levator ani muscles, and lateral to them the ischio-rectal fossae. These are large pads of fatty tissue which lie between the anal canal and the lower part of the lateral pelvic walls.

The blood supply is received from the superior, middle and inferior haemorrhoidal arteries and the median sacral artery. The veins drain in a similar manner, those forming the superior haemorrhoidal vein being the site of origin of internal haemorrhoids.

The lymph drainage is into the internal iliac glands, the anus itself draining with the skin of the perineum into the inguinal glands.

The nerve supply of the upper half of the anal canal is derived through the Lee-Frankenhäuser plexus and consists of sympathetic and para-sympathetic fibres. The lower half is supplied by a somatic nerve, the inferior haemorrhoidal, which is a branch of the pudendal nerve.

The Physiology of Defaecation

Defaecation is normally a voluntary act under the control of the will. When faeces enter the rectum from the pelvic colon by the action of peristalsis they give rise to the desire to defaecate. During the act the pelvic colon and rectum contract by para-sympathetic action, and increased intra-abdominal pressure expels the faeces. The anal canal, which is normally closed, opens through relaxation of the sphincters to allow the faeces to pass, and this expansion is permitted by the soft ischio-rectal fossae. At the end of the act the anus is raised by the levator ani muscles which surround the anal canal (hence their name), the sphincters become contracted, and the rectum is then closed to the exterior.

THE PELVIC FLOOR

The soft tissues which fill the outlet of the pelvis comprise what is

...e pelvic floor. It is apparent that in the erect attitude ...an beings have adopted, the weight of the abdominal ...sts on the floor of the pelvis, and in consequence this is a ...ucture made up of fascia and muscles. At the same time, ...c outlet is the exit from the body whereby the contents of the bladder, uterus and rectum are evacuated; accordingly the pelvic floor is pierced by the urethra, vagina and anal canal.

1. The Muscles of the Pelvic Floor

It is convenient first to consider the muscles which comprise the pelvic floor. They consist of two deep muscles, the levatores ani, and a superficial group of muscles known as the superficial perineal muscles. The levator ani muscles and the pelvic fascia which clothes them above and below are sometimes referred to as the pelvic diaphragm.

A. The Levator Ani Muscles

These are two powerful muscles, 3 to 5 mm. in thickness, lying on either side of the pelvis. They arise from the circumference of the true

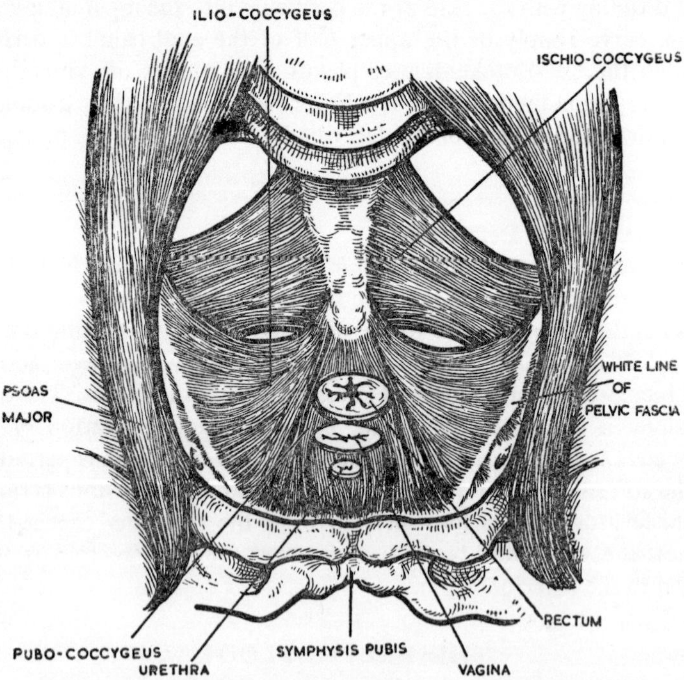

Figure 16. View from above of the levator ani muscles

pelvis and converge towards the midline, with a concave upper and convex lower surface, to be inserted into the perineal body, the anal canal, the ano-coccygeal body, the coccyx and the lower end of the sacrum. They consist of three parts, each one of which is associated with one of the constituent bones of the innominate bone:

(i) *The pubo-coccygeus* arises from the back of the bodies of the pubic bones. The muscle fibres sweep posteriorly below the bladder, on either side of the urethra and the lowest third of the vagina, to enter the perineal body. Here some fibres cross from side to side and form the deep half of the perineal body: others pass on and are inserted into the wall of the anal canal, whilst others form a loop around this structure known as the ano-rectal sling. The longest fibres gain insertions into the ano-coccygeal body and the coccyx.

(ii) *The ilio-coccygeus* takes origin from the iliac part of the pelvic brim in lower animals, but in human beings the origin is different and the muscle fibres arise from the fascia covering the obturator internus muscle. The site of origin of the ilio-coccygeus is marked by a thick white line, known as the 'white line of pelvic fascia'. The fibres sweep downwards and inwards and are inserted into the ano-coccygeal body and the coccyx.

(iii) *The ischio-coccygeus* is situated in front of the sacro-spinous ligament, and is sometimes referred to as a separate muscle, the coccygeus muscle. Its fibres arise behind the ilio-coccygeus from the spine of the ischium and pass downwards and inwards to be inserted into the coccyx and the lowest piece of the sacrum.

It can thus be understood that in the upright position the levator ani muscles form a hammock across the pelvis which carries the weight of the abdominal organs, and which is pierced by the urethra, vagina and anal canal. A space exists behind the muscle corresponding to the position of the greater sciatic notch, which on account of the tilting of the pelvis when the patient stands erect, is really the posterior wall of the pelvis rather than its floor. This space is filled by the piriformis muscle which passes from the sacrum through the greater sciatic notch on its way to gain insertion into the greater trochanter of the femur. Nerves from the sacral plexus also leave the pelvis through the notch with the piriformis muscle.

The function of the levator ani muscles is to form a muscular diaphragm to support the pelvic viscera, and to counteract any increase in the intra-abdominal pressure. It thus supports the bladder and vagina, and constricts the lower end of this latter organ; when it contracts the ano-rectal sling pulls the rectum, at the point where it becomes continuous with the anal canal, towards the pubic bones and so kinks the gut. It also closes the anal canal, and lifts up the anus after defaecation thereby assisting in the expulsion of faeces. During labour it plays some part in guiding the foetus in its passage through the birth canal.

The attachment of the levator ani to the coccyx has already been noted. In lower animals where the coccyx forms the tail, the levator ani functions as a tail-moving muscle. Thus a happy dog wags his tail by alternately contracting his ischio-coccygei, whilst a naughty dog slinks away with his tail drawn down by his pubo-coccygei.

The levator ani muscle is supplied by the pudendal nerve and the ourth sacral nerve.

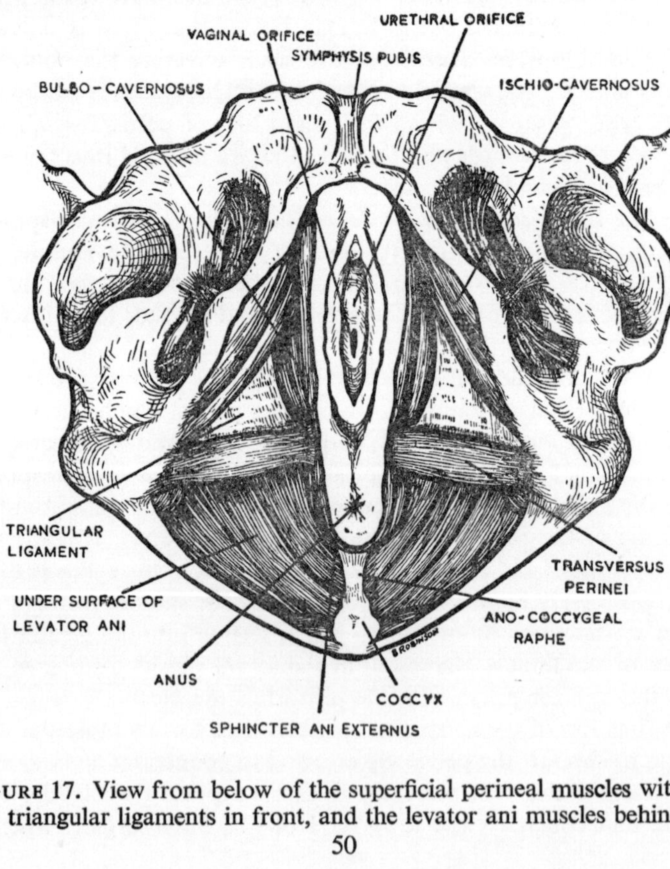

FIGURE 17. View from below of the superficial perineal muscles with the triangular ligaments in front, and the levator ani muscles behind

B. THE SUPERFICIAL PERINEAL MUSCLES

These muscles lie in the pelvic outlet on the under surface of the anterior part of the levator ani muscles, forming the superficial half of the perineal body and surrounding the anal and vaginal orifices. On either side of the anal canal below the posterior part of the levator muscles lie the ischio-rectal fossae. The superficial perineal muscles are important as they are liable to injury during childbirth. They may be described as follows:

(i) *The external sphincter of the anus* surrounds the anal canal, lying below the internal sphincter and the levatores ani. Anteriorly it enters into the formation of the perineal body, where it is attached to other superficial perineal muscles at a point known as the central point of the perineum. Posteriorly some of its fibres are attached to the tip of the coccyx. Its function is to close the lumen of the anal canal.

(ii) *The transverse perineal muscles* take origin from the ischial tuberosities and pass transversely inwards to meet their fellow of the opposite side and other perineal muscles in the central point of the

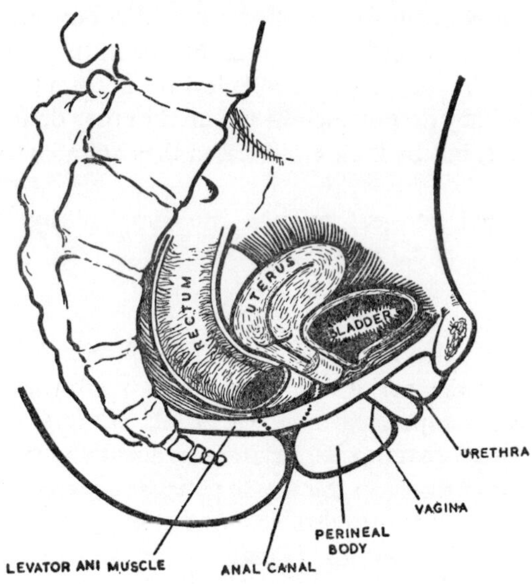

FIGURE 18. Lateral view of pelvis showing how the levator ani muscles form part of the pelvic floor. Note how they are pierced by the urethra, vagina and anal canal

perineum. They consist of superficial and deep portions—the deep muscle is enclosed between the layers of the triangular ligament. These muscles fix the position of the perineal body and help to support the lower part of the vagina.

(iii) *The bulbo-cavernosus* (or *bulbo-spongiosus*) *muscles* arise from the central point of the perineum and pass forwards around the vagina, lying superficial to Bartholin's glands and the vestibular bulbs and deep to the labia. They are inserted into the corpora cavernosa of the clitoris in the upper part of the pubic arch. The action of these muscles is to diminish the size of the vaginal orifice and to cause engorgement of the clitoris, but they are small muscles and their action is weak.

(iv) *The ischio-cavernosus muscles* arise from the ischial tuberosities and pass upwards and inwards along the pubic arch to gain insertion into the corpora cavernosa of the clitoris. Their function is to cause engorgement of the clitoris.

(v) *The membranous sphincter of the urethra.* Although from the obstetrical point of view this muscle is not situated in the perineum, it is anatomically allied to the other superficial perineal muscles. It lies between the layers of the triangular ligament. Its fibres arise from one pubic bone and pass above and below the urethra to the opposite pubic bone; as they do not encircle the urethra they do not constitute a true sphincter, but by their contraction they are able to occlude its lumen.

The superficial perineal muscles are supplied by the perineal branch of the pudendal nerve.

The Triangular Ligament

This structure (also known as the inferior fascia of the urogenital diaphragm and the perineal membrane) is really the deep fascia which invests these perineal muscles. It fills in the triangular space between the bulbo-cavernosus, ischio-cavernosus and transverse perineal muscles, and the deep transverse perineal muscles and the membranous sphincter of the urethra lie between its layers. It is pierced by the urethra and the vagina and helps to maintain them in their normal positions.

The Perineal Body

The constituent parts of this structure have now been described. It is a fibro-muscular pyramid situated between the lowest third of the vagina in front, the anal canal behind and the ischial tuberosities laterally. Its deeper half consists of fibres from the levatores ani which cross from side to side between the vagina and the anal canal, whilst its lower half is made up of the superficial perineal muscles. The centre of its lowest part, to which many of the superficial perineal muscles converge, is known as the central point of the perineum. It is covered by superficial fascia and skin.

A superficial perineal laceration occurring during childbirth may tear the skin and the bulbo-cavernosus and transverse perineal muscles; a deeper tear may involve the levatores ani in addition, whilst a third-degree tear lacerates the external sphincter of the anus. Damage to the membranous sphincter of the urethra during labour disturbs the support of the bladder neck, and leads to the development of stress incontinence.

2. The Fascia of the Pelvic Floor

On the upper surface of the levator ani muscles are situated the bladder and ureters, the upper two-thirds of the vagina, the uterus with its appendages, and the rectum, together with the blood-vessels, lymphatics and nerves which supply them. These organs are embedded in a layer of loose areolar tissue which invests them, fills the spaces between them, and extends from the pelvic peritoneum above to the levator ani muscles below. This is known as the pelvic fascia. It consists of two parts:

A. The Parietal Pelvic Fascia

The pelvic wall is lined by a layer of this fascia, called the parietal pelvic fascia, part of which is thickened to form the 'white line of pelvic fascia', which gives origin to the ilio-coccygeal portion of the levator ani muscle. Below the levator ani it passes down the side wall of the pelvis and lines the lateral wall of the ischio-rectal fossa, whilst in front of this it fuses with the triangular ligament. Anteriorly, the parietal pelvic fascia covers part of the pubic bones, and posteriorly, it clothes the piriformis and is attached to the sacrum. Above, it is continuous with the fasciae of the abdominal wall.

B. The Visceral Pelvic Fascia

The pelvic organs are invested by the visceral layer of pelvic fascia. The part of the fascia which surrounds the bladder and rectum is thickened to form the supporting ligaments of these organs, whilst the fascia investing the upper parts of the vagina and cervix contains muscle fibres and forms the supporting ligaments of the uterus as already described. This portion is sometimes called the parametrium. The fascia also lies between the two peritoneal layers which form the broad ligaments. As the ureters, vessels and nerves pass from the walls of the pelvis to the pelvic organs, they ramify in this layer of visceral pelvic fascia. It also covers the lower surface of the levator ani muscles, where it is known as the anal fascia.

The structures which form the pelvic floor from above downwards are thus:

i. The pelvic peritoneum.

ii. The visceral layer of pelvic fascia, condensed in places to form the supporting ligaments of the pelvic viscera.

iii. The levator ani muscles.

iv. The anal fascia.

v. The superficial perineal muscles and the triangular ligament.

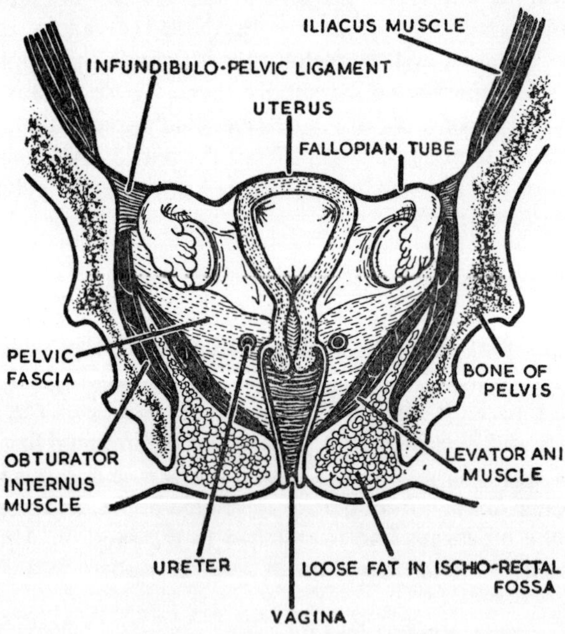

FIGURE 19. Transverse section of pelvis to show the formation of the pelvic floor. Note relation of the visceral pelvic fascia, the levator ani muscles and the ischio-rectal fossae

vi. The superficial fascia and the ischio-rectal fossae.
vii. The skin.

Other Muscles of the Pelvis

1. *The piriformis muscles.* These are two in number and occupy the posterior part of the pelvic wall. They arise from the anterior surface of the second, third and fourth sacral vertebrae, and pass out of the pelvis through the greater sciatic notch to be inserted into the greater trochanter of the femur. They are supplied by branches from the first and second sacral nerves, and their action is to rotate the thighs laterally.

2. *The obturator internus muscles.* These form part of the side walls of the pelvis and are covered by parietal pelvic fascia. They arise from the inner surfaces of the pubis, ischium, ilium and obturator membrane. The muscle fibres converge towards the lesser sciatic notch where they leave the pelvis to be inserted into the greater trochanter of the femur. Their nerve of supply is a branch from the sacral plexus and their function also is to rotate the thighs laterally.

3. *The iliacus muscles.* These are two flat triangular muscles, each of which arises from an iliac fossa. The fibres pass downwards and gradually converge as they lie over the pelvic brim and pass under the inguinal ligament. They are inserted into the tendon of the psoas major muscle. The iliacus is supplied by a branch from the femoral nerve.

4. *The psoas major muscles.* These are two muscles which arise mainly from the bodies and transverse processes of the lumbar vertebrae and pass downwards across the pelvic brim, below the inguinal ligament and in front of the hip joint, where they form a tendon. This is joined by the fibres of the iliacus muscle, and is inserted into the lesser trochanter of the femur. The nerve supply is received from the second, third, and fourth lumbar nerves.

These two muscles are sometimes considered to form a single functional unit known as the ilio-psoas muscle. Its function is to flex the thigh and, acting in conjunction with the gluteal muscles in the erect attitude, it helps to stabilize the hip joint.

THE ARTERIES OF THE PELVIS

Four large arteries are mainly responsible for the blood supply to the pelvic organs, namely the two ovarian arteries and the two internal iliac (or hypogastric) arteries. Also present are the fibrosed remains of two large arteries which function during foetal life—the obliterated hypogastric arteries.

1. The Ovarian Arteries

These arise from the abdominal aorta, just below the level of the renal arteries.

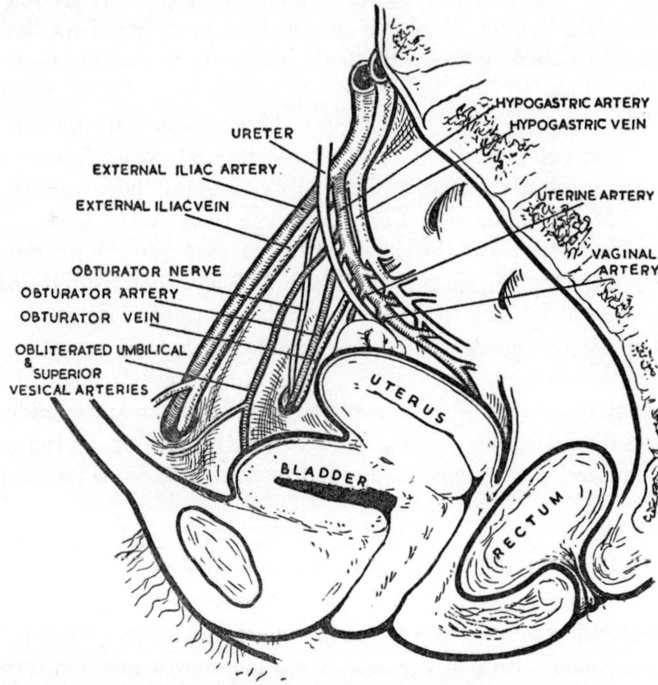

FIGURE 20. Side view of pelvis, showing arteries and veins

COURSE

Each artery passes obliquely downwards and outwards behind the peritoneum and reaches the pelvic brim, where it crosses the external iliac artery and vein and enters the true pelvis. It then passes through the infundibulo-pelvic ligament, enters the broad ligament of the uterus and passes through the mesovarium into the ovary. One or more branches supply the Fallopian tube, whilst another passes down alongside the uterus to unite with the uterine artery of the same side.

2. The Internal Iliac Arteries

Each artery begins in front of the upper part of the sacro-iliac joint, where the common iliac artery terminates by dividing into the external and internal iliac arteries. The external iliac vessel passes below the inguinal ligament and enters the thigh, being the main vessel of supply to the lower limb, whilst the internal iliac artery is the chief source of supply to all the pelvic viscera.

COURSE

The internal iliac artery, which is only about two inches (5 cm.) long, passes downwards into the pelvis in front of the sacro-iliac joint to reach the upper part of the greater sciatic notch.

RELATIONS

During its course it has the following relations:

Posterior. The internal iliac vein, the lumbo-sacral nerve trunk and the sacro-iliac joint.

Anterior. The ureter and the ovarian fossa.

Lateral. The pelvic wall.

Medial. The pelvic peritoneum.

BRANCHES

Opposite the upper border of the sciatic notch the internal iliac artery divides into a large number of branches:

(i) *The uterine artery* runs medially from the lateral pelvic wall in the visceral pelvic fascia on the upper surface of the levator ani muscle, crossing above the ureter by the side of the cervix, to reach the uterus at the level of the internal os. It then ascends alongside the corpus of the uterus, between the layers of the broad ligament, in a winding and tortuous manner. When it reaches the cornu it turns laterally and joins with a branch of the ovarian artery below the Fallopian tube. It gives off branches which supply the lower end of the ureter, the cervix and the vagina and sends numerous branches into the body of the uterus and the Fallopian tube. Those entering the myometrium pass in a circular direction towards the midline where they anastomose with those of the opposite side. They constitute the coronary arteries.

(ii) *The vaginal artery* passes medially in the visceral pelvic fascia to reach the vagina, which it supplies. It anastomoses with branches from the uterine arteries above, and sometimes forms large vessels which pass down the anterior and posterior vaginal walls in the midline. These are known as the azygos arteries of the vagina.

(iii) *The superior vesical artery* runs forwards to the bladder where it supplies its upper part.

(iv) *The inferior vesical artery* passes forwards to the base of the bladder, which it supplies along with the lower end of the ureter.

(v) *The middle haemorrhoidal artery* passes medially to supply the rectum.

(vi) *The internal pudendal artery* leaves the pelvis through the greater sciatic notch, crosses the ischial spine and then enters the ischio-rectal fossa through the lesser sciatic notch. It then runs in a tunnel (Alcock's canal) in the parietal pelvic fascia in the lateral wall of the fossa above the ischial tuberosity, and passes along the pubic arch, supplying the anal canal (by a branch called the inferior haemorrhoidal artery), the perineal body, the labia, the vestibular bulbs and the clitoris. Throughout most of its course it is accompanied by the pudendal nerve.

(vii) Other branches are the obturator, superior and inferior gluteals, the ilio-lumbar and the lateral sacral arteries. These in the main are arteries which supply muscles outside the pelvis.

3. The Obliterated Hypogastric Arteries

During foetal life, when the legs are relatively small, the major part of the foetal blood passes from the aorta and common iliac arteries into the internal iliac arteries, which carry it up the anterior abdominal wall to the umbilicus. During this time these arteries are known as the hypogastric arteries, and after passing through the umbilicus they enter the cord and become the umbilical arteries.

At birth, when the foetal circulation changes into that of the adult, modifications occur in the foetal hypogastric arteries, as described in Chapter 6. The proximal portions remain patent and become the superior vesical arteries; the distal portions are changed into fibrous ligaments, which are then known as the obliterated hypogastric arteries. These can be traced on each side of the pelvic wall as ligaments running from the superior vesical arteries on to the anterior abdominal wall outside the peritoneum. They then pass in a converging manner up to the umbilicus, which they enter alongside the urachus.

4. Branches from the Femoral Artery

The superficial and deep external pudendal branches of the femoral artery ascend from the upper part of the thigh and supply the labia majora.

THE VEINS OF THE PELVIS

These are very similar in their distribution to the arteries which they accompany, the blood from the pelvic organs draining away chiefly by the ovarian and internal iliac veins.

1. The Ovarian Veins

These are formed within the broad ligament by branches from the ovary, uterus and Fallopian tube which unite and form a plexus; this passes into the infundibulo-pelvic ligament, where it is called the pampiniform plexus. Finally a single ovarian vein is formed on each side which passes upwards behind the peritoneum and ends in a

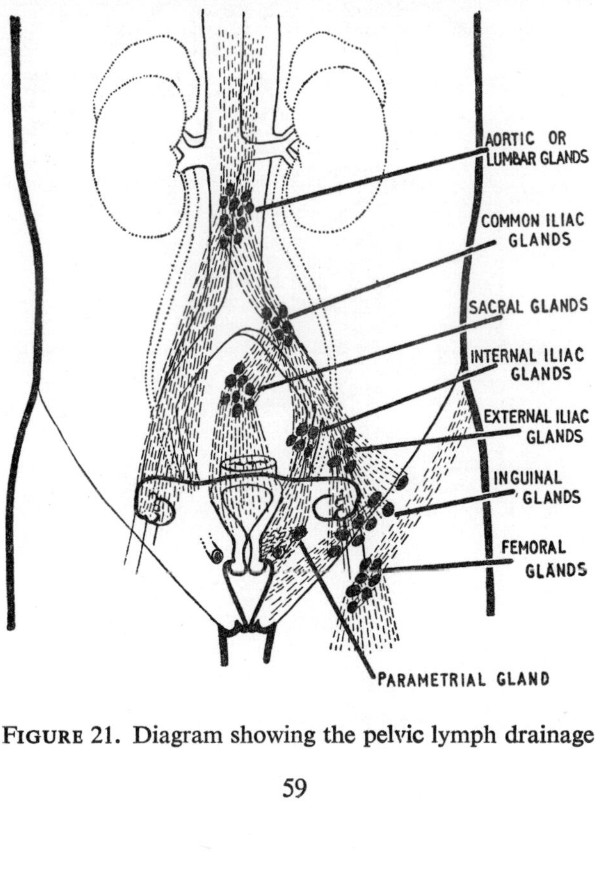

FIGURE 21. Diagram showing the pelvic lymph drainage

different manner on the two sides. On the right, the ovarian vein opens into the inferior vena cava below the renal veins, whilst on the left, the ovarian vein opens into the left renal vein itself.

2. The Internal Iliac Veins

These are made up of tributaries which originate in large plexuses around the vagina, uterus, and bladder, and then unite to form veins which correspond to the branches of the internal iliac arteries. They pass up posterior to the internal iliac arteries, and join with the external iliac veins coming from the legs to form the common iliac veins. These unite to form the inferior vena cava.

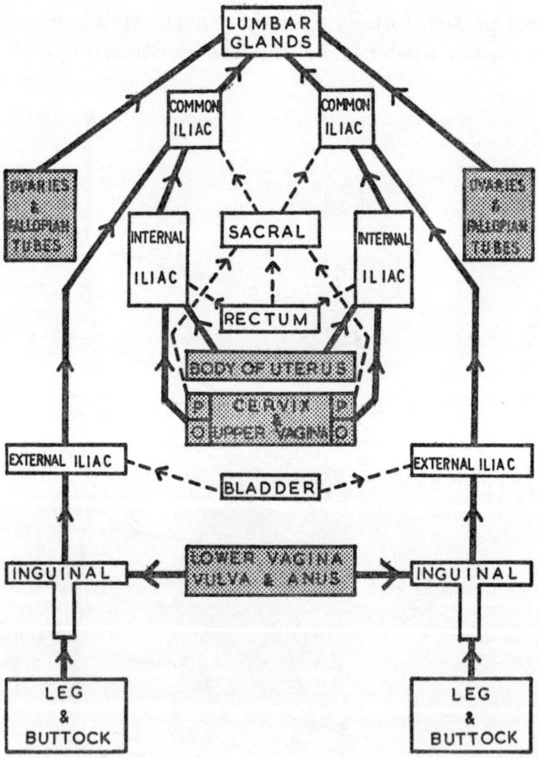

FIGURE 22. Schematic representation of the lymph drainage of the pelvis

THE LYMPHATICS OF THE PELVIS

There are numerous groups of lymphatic glands which receive lymph from the pelvic organs and transmit it to further groups on its way to reach the receptaculum chyli.

The most important groups are as follows:

(i) *The inguinal group* consists of a horizontal set lying along the inguinal ligament of the groin, and a vertical set passing for about 4½ inches (11·4 cm.) down into the thigh alongside the saphenous and femoral veins. The former group drains the vulva, including Bartholin's gland, the anus, the lowest third of the vagina and the perineal body, whilst the latter group receives lymph from the buttocks and lower limbs. A small lymphatic vessel from the fundus of the uterus passes along the round ligament to join the horizontal group of glands.

(ii) *The external iliac group* lies alongside the external iliac vessels and receives lymph from the inguinal glands in addition to directly draining the bladder.

(iii) *The parametrial gland* is only sometimes present, and then is placed in the parametrium alongside the cervix, close to where the uterine artery and vein cross the ureter. It drains lymph from the cervix.

(iv) *The obturator group* lies in the obturator fossa, in the upper part of the foramen ovale, and receives lymph from the cervix and bladder.

(v) *The internal iliac group* is situated along the course of the internal iliac vessels, and receives lymph mainly from the body and cervix of the uterus, the upper two-thirds of the vagina, the urethra, the rectum and the anal canal. These glands also drain the parametrial and obturator glands.

(vi) *The sacral group* is placed lateral to the rectum in the hollow of the sacrum, and receives lymph from the uterus, upper vagina and rectum.

(vii) *The common iliac glands* surround the common iliac vessels, and receive lymph from the internal and external iliac groups and the sacral group.

(viii) *The lumbar glands* directly drain the ovaries and Fallopian tubes, and also receive lymph from the common iliac glands before transmitting it to the receptaculum chyli.

THE NERVES OF THE PELVIS

The pelvic organs are supplied by two sets of nerves, the sympathetic and para-sympathetic systems, whose functions are mutually antagonistic. The sympathetic nerves inhibit muscles which expel visceral contents, cause sphincters to contract and vessels to undergo constriction. The para-sympathetic fibres have the opposite effect and cause visceral organs to expel their contents, sphincters to relax, and vessels to become dilated.

The Sympathetic Supply

The sympathetic supply in the main is the pelvic continuation of the large abdominal sympathetic plexuses, the most important of which are the coeliac or solar plexus, the aortic plexus and the renal plexuses.

The aortic plexus is continued below the level of the bifurcation of the aorta as a large network of nerves which lies in front of the last lumbar vertebra and the promontory of the sacrum. This is sometimes called the 'pre-sacral nerve', and it is joined by branches from the lumbar sympathetic chains. As it passes downwards it divides into two branches which terminate in plexuses lying in the floor of the pouch of Douglas on each side of the rectum, in the region of the utero-sacral ligaments. This network also receives fibres from the para-sympathetic system and is known as the plexus of Lee-Frankenhäuser. From here nerves pass to all the pelvic viscera.

The ovarian plexus consists of sympathetic fibres derived from the renal and coeliac plexuses which accompany the ovarian vessels through the infundibulo-pelvic ligaments to supply the ovaries and the Fallopian tubes.

The Para-sympathetic Supply

The para-sympathetic nerves are known as the nervi erigentes, and are derived from the second and third sacral segments. The fibres emerge from the anterior sacral foramina corresponding to these segments of the cord and enter the plexus of Lee-Frankenhäuser, subsequently to be distributed to all the pelvic viscera.

Somatic Nerves

Many of the nerves which supply the lower limbs pass through the pelvis to reach their destinations. Large nerve trunks emerge through the four anterior sacral foramina on each side, and divide and unite to form the sacral plexus. This lies on the posterior wall of the pelvic cavity in front of the piriformis muscle, and is joined from above by the lumbo-sacral nerve trunk (derived from the fourth and fifth lumbar nerves) which passes in front of the sacro-iliac joint to reach it. The terminal branches of the plexus leave the pelvis through the greater sciatic notch in company with the piriformis muscle behind the posterior part of the levator ani.

Some of these nerves are of importance to obstetricians:

1. The pudendal nerve, which is a branch of the sacral plexus, leaves the pelvis through the greater sciatic notch, crosses the ischial spine and re-enters the pelvis through the lesser sciatic notch to pass into Alcock's canal in the lateral wall of the ischio-rectal fossa above the ischial tuberosity. It then gives off the inferior haemorrhoidal nerve which supplies the anal canal and its sphincters. Its terminal branches, the perineal nerve and the dorsal nerve of the clitoris, then run along the pubic arch and supply the superficial perineal muscles, the lower part of the levator ani and the skin of the vulva. The internal pudendal vessels accompany this nerve and its branches throughout their course.

Regional anaesthesia may be induced for forceps delivery or breech delivery by injecting a local anaesthetic solution into Alcock's canal. This causes anaesthesia of the vulva, lower vagina and perineum, which are supplied by sensory branches from the pudendal nerve.

Complete anaesthesia, however, is only achieved if three other nerves which supply the skin of the vulva are also infiltrated with the solution. These are:

(a) The ilio-inguinal nerve, which emerges from the inguinal canal with the round ligament of the uterus and supplies the skin of the anterior part of the vulva.

(b) The genital branch of the genito-femoral nerve, whose course and distribution are similar.

(c) The perineal branch of the posterior cutaneous nerve of the thigh, which supplies the skin of the posterior part of the vulva.

2. A branch from the fourth sacral nerve passes directly to supply the upper part of the levator ani muscles and part of the external anal sphincter.

3. The lumbo-sacral trunk may be injured during difficult labours,

as it lies in front of the sacro-iliac joint. The peroneal and anterior tibial muscles which are supplied by this nerve trunk in the leg may then be paralysed, giving rise to the condition known as foot-drop.

CHAPTER 3

The Anatomy of the Bony Pelvis

A knowledge of the bony pelvis is of great importance to the student of midwifery, for during birth the foetus has to traverse the relatively unyielding ring which it forms on its passage from the uterus to the vulva. It is composed of the two innominate bones, which comprise its anterior and lateral parts, together with the sacrum and coccyx, which are placed posteriorly. Each innominate bone is formed by the fusion of three bones, the ilium, ischium and pubis.

THE BONES OF THE PELVIS

1. The Ilium

This is made up of a relatively flat plate of bone above, and part of the acetabulum below. It has the following characteristics:

(i) The external aspect of the bony plate is gently curved and has a roughened surface to which are attached the gluteal muscles of the buttock.

(ii) The greater part of the inner aspect is smooth and concave, forming the iliac fossa. In life a muscle originates from here, the iliacus, which forms a soft platform on which the abdominal viscera rest.

(iii) The ridge which surmounts these two surfaces is known as the iliac crest. This is shaped like an elongated letter S, and serves for the attachment of the muscles of the abdominal wall. Anteriorly the crest ends in the anterior superior iliac spine, a bony prominence which can readily be palpated under the skin, whilst posteriorly it ends in the posterior superior iliac spine, a point which is marked in the living subject by a dimple at the level of the second sacral vertebra.

If the back be inspected these dimples will be seen to form the lateral angles of a flat diamond-shaped area, the upper point of which corresponds approximately to the spine of the fifth lumbar vertebra, whilst the lowest point lies in the upper end of the gluteal cleft. This area is known as the rhomboid of Michaelis.

(iv) Below the anterior superior iliac spine is another bony prominence, the anterior inferior iliac spine, whilst posteriorly is similarly situated the posterior inferior iliac spine.

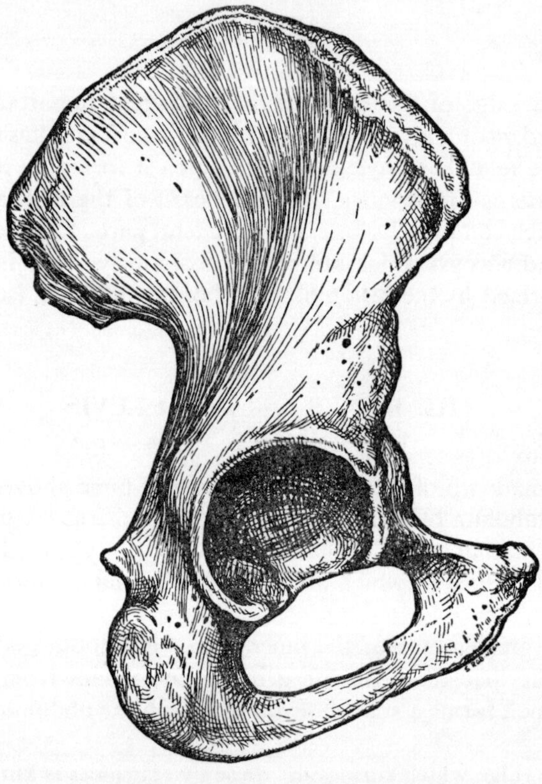

FIGURE 23. Lateral view of the right innominate bone

(v) At its lowermost part the ilium forms two-fifths of the acetabulum, where it fuses with the ischium and pubis.

(vi) Behind the acetabulum, the ilium forms the upper part of a large notch, the greater sciatic notch, through which pass the piriformis muscle and the nerves of the sacral plexus, on their way from the front of the sacrum into the thigh.

(vii) On the inner aspect of the bone, the iliac fossa is bounded below by a prominent ridge, which is the iliac part of the ilio-pectineal line. At a lower level the ilium enters into the formation of the side wall of the true pelvis, where it forms part of the floor of the acetabulum. Anteriorly the ilio-pectineal line swells into a bony prominence, at the point where the ilium fuses with the superior ramus of the pubis, to form the ilio-pectineal eminence.

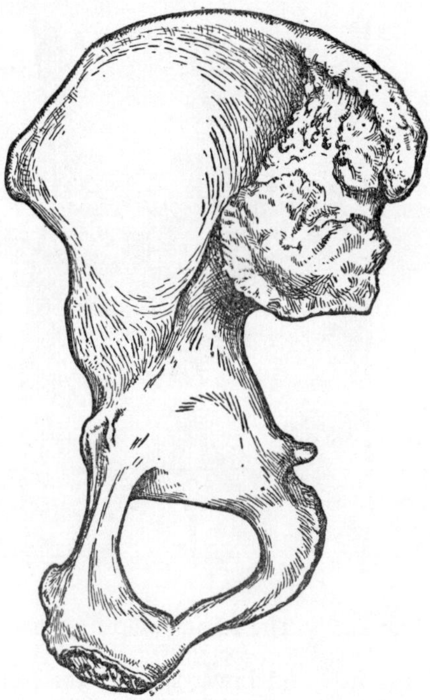

FIGURE 24. Medial view of the right innominate bone

(viii) Posterior to the ilio-pectineal line, and above the greater sciatic notch, is a roughened area where the ilium articulates with the sacrum to form the sacro-iliac joint. The tough supporting ligaments of this joint are attached to the bone behind the articular surface.

2. The Ischium

The ischium is the lowest of the constituent bones of the innominate bone, and is formed by the following parts:

(i) The head forms the lowest two-fifths of the acetabulum, where it fuses with the ilium and pubis.

(ii) Below the acetabulum a thick buttress of bone passes downwards and terminates in the ischial tuberosity. It is this part of the pelvis on which the weight of the body rests when sitting; it gives origin to the hamstring muscles of the thigh and is covered by a large bursa.

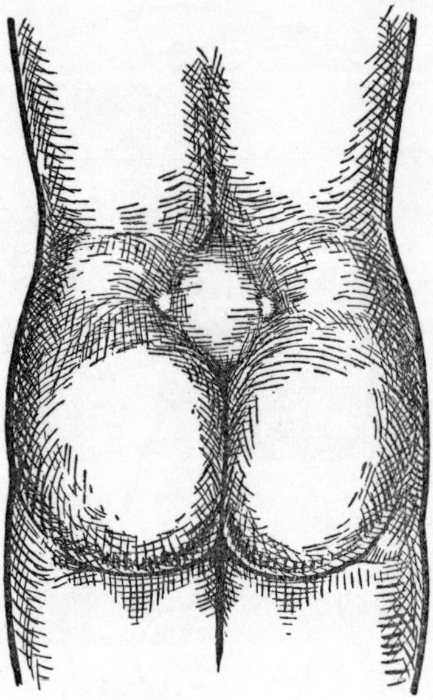

FIGURE 25. The Rhomboid of Michaelis

(iii) Passing upwards and inwards from the ischial tuberosity a small shaft of the ischium becomes continuous with the inferior ramus of the pubis, so forming the pubic arch.

(iv) The ischium thus forms the lower boundary of a large foramen, the obturator foramen or foramen ovale.

(v) On its internal aspect the ischium forms the side wall of the true pelvis. Protruding inwards from its posterior edge, about two inches above the tuberosity, is a conspicuous projection known as the ischial spine. This separates the greater sciatic notch above, which transmits the piriformis muscle and the branches of the sacral plexus, from the lesser sciatic notch below, through which the tendon of the obturator internus muscle leaves the pelvis on its way to find insertion into the greater trochanter of the femur. The lesser notch is thus situated between the ischial spine above and the ischial tuberosity below.

3. The Pubis

This is the smallest of the three bones forming the innominate bone and it is the only one which articulates with its fellow of the opposite side. Each pubic bone presents the following features:

(i) The body of the pubis is square-shaped, with its medial side entering with that of its fellow into the formation of a joint known as the symphysis pubis.

(ii) The upper surface of the body forms a crest, the pubic crest, which ends laterally in the pubic tubercle.

(iii) Laterally the superior ramus passes to the acetabulum, of which it forms one-fifth, where it fuses with the ilium and ischium. Its junction with the ilium passes through the ilio-pectineal eminence. Its upper surface is marked by a ridge which runs from the pubic tubercle to the ilio-pectineal eminence. This is the forward extension of the ilio-pectineal line on to the pubis and is known as the pubic part of the ilio-pectineal line. The superior ramus completes the upper boundary of the foramen ovale.

(iv) Below the body of the pubis, the inferior ramus passes downwards and outwards to join the ischium, so forming the upper part of the pubic arch.

These three bones are each formed from pre-existing cartilage, and their separate ossification centres become fused together about the age of puberty. Ossification in the pelvis, however, is not completed before the age of twenty-five.

4. The Sacrum

The sacrum is situated in the posterior part of the pelvis, where it articulates with the iliac portions of the two innominate bones at the sacro-iliac joints. It presents the following salient features:

(i) It consists usually of five sacral vertebrae which have become fused into one solid mass of bone. The anterior surface is smooth, and is concave from above downwards and slightly so from side to side, forming what is known as the hollow of the sacrum.

(ii) The first sacral vertebra overhangs the sacral hollow, and the central point of its upper projecting margin is known as the promontory of the sacrum.

(iii) The anterior branches of the first four pairs of sacral nerves emerge from the sacral canal through eight large foramina situated in the hollow of the sacrum. After forming the sacral plexus these nerves mostly pass through the greater sciatic notch into the thigh.

(iv) The posterior surface of the sacrum is rough and irregular and serves for the attachment of the ligaments and muscles of the back. Eight small foramina are present, through which the small posterior branches of the sacral nerves emerge to supply the skin of the buttocks and the muscles of the lower part of the back.

(v) Passing longitudinally through the centre of the bone, but nearer to its posterior surface, is the sacral canal. This contains the sacral and coccygeal nerves derived from the spinal cord.

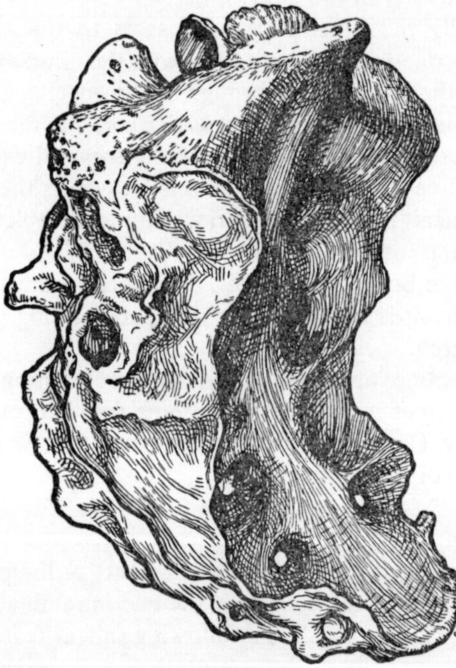

FIGURE 26. Lateral view of the sacrum

(vi) The sacral canal opens on to the posterior surface of the bone opposite the fifth sacral vertebra, between two projections known as the sacral cornua. When a caudal block is induced during labour, the local anaesthetic solution is injected between these two sacral cornua into the lower part of the sacral canal. The dura mater terminates opposite the second sacral vertebra, and the anaesthetic paralyses the nerves lying in the sacral canal below this level.

(vii) On its upper surface is a smooth oval area where the sacrum articulates with the fifth lumbar vertebra forming the lumbo-sacral joint. The lateral masses of bone on either side of this articular surface are known as the wings of the sacrum, or the sacral alae.

(viii) Opposite the first two sacral vertebrae the lateral aspects of the bone are relatively smooth where they enter into the formation of the sacro-iliac joints.

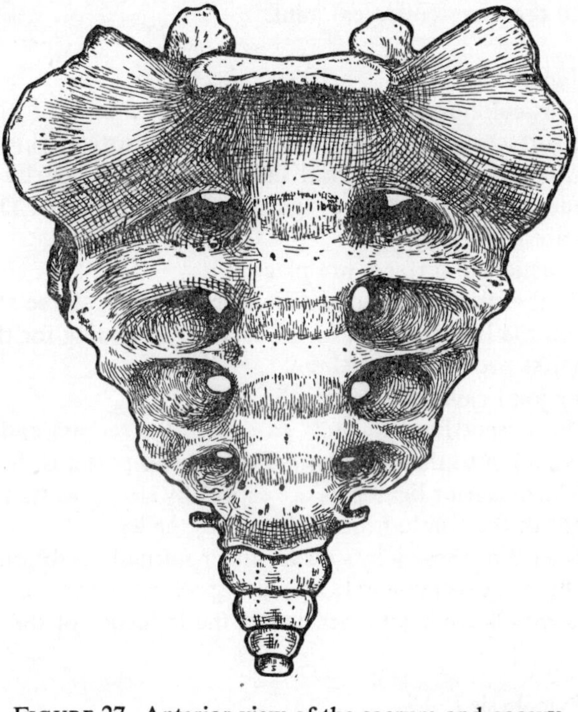

FIGURE 27. Anterior view of the sacrum and coccyx

(ix) The lower margin of the sacrum forms a small smooth surface where it articulates with the coccyx at the sacro-coccygeal joint.

5. The Coccyx

This small bone consists of four fused coccygeal vertebrae. It is triangular in shape with its base uppermost.

(i) The first coccygeal vertebra articulates with the lower end of the sacrum at the sacro-coccygeal joint. It contains two small cornua which project upwards towards the sacral cornua.

(ii) The remaining three vertebrae are mere rudimentary nodules of bone; they are smooth on their inner surface where they support the rectum, whilst to their lowermost tip is attached the external anal sphincter and the ano-coccygeal body.

THE PELVIC JOINTS

These are four in number, the two sacro-iliac joints the symphysis pubis and the sacro-coccygeal joint.

1. The Sacro-Iliac Joints

These articulations have the customary formation of joints with articular surfaces covered with cartilage on the articulating bones, a joint cavity filled with synovial fluid, a capsule lined by synovial membrane, and surrounding tough supporting ligaments. Their main features are as follows:

(i) The articular surfaces are placed:

(a) on the inner surface of the ilium above the greater sciatic notch;

(b) on the lateral aspect of the sacrum, extending for the length of the first two sacral vertebrae.

(ii) The joint cavity is very small.

(iii) The supporting ligaments pass from the sacrum and the fifth lumbar vertebra to the ilium both anterior and posterior to the joint cavity. The posterior ligaments are especially strong as they transmit the weight of the trunk, head and arms to the legs.

Movements at these joints occur under normal conditions but are very slight. They increase in range during pregnancy and labour when the ligaments become softened under the influence of the hormone relaxin.

2. The Symphysis Pubis

This joint consists of an oval disc of fibro-cartilage, about $1\frac{1}{2}$ inches (3·8 cm.) long, which is interposed between the bodies of the two pubic bones. It sometimes contains a small cavity, which is not lined by synovial membrane.

The symphysis is reinforced by supporting ligaments which pass from one pubic bone to the other in front, behind, above and below the disc of cartilage.

3. The Sacro-Coccygeal Joint

This small joint is situated between the lower border of the sacrum and the upper border of the coccyx. The articular surfaces of the bones are smooth and an intervertebral disc of cartilage lies between them, with supporting ligaments placed in front, behind and laterally. Sometimes a small joint cavity lined with synovial membrane is present.

Slight backward and forward movements of the coccyx on the lower end of the sacrum occur normally; the backward movement is greatly increased during labour at the time of the actual birth of the head.

THE PELVIC LIGAMENTS

The pelvic ligaments of importance to the midwife are as follows:

1. The supporting ligaments of the pelvic joints already described.

2. The sacro-tuberous ligament, which is a strong ligament passing from the posterior superior iliac spine and the lateral borders of the sacrum and the coccyx to the ischial tuberosity. It bridges across the greater and lesser sciatic notches.

3. The sacro-spinous ligament, which is another strong ligament passing from the side of the sacrum and coccyx across the greater sciatic notch to the ischial spine. It lies in front of the sacro-tuberous ligament.

4. The inguinal ligament (Poupart's ligament), which consists of the lower border of the tendon of the external oblique muscle of the anterior abdominal wall. It runs from the anterior superior iliac spine to the pubic tubercle forming the groin.

5. The lacunar ligament (Gimbernat's ligament) is a small ligament which occupies the angle between the inner end of the inguinal ligament and the upper part of the pubic bone.

6. The obturator membrane, which is a ligament closing the foramen ovale, with the exception of a small area in its upper part which transmits the obturator vessels and nerve and contains the obturator lymphatic glands.

THE PELVIS AS A WHOLE

Although it is valuable to possess a knowledge of the constituent bones and joints of the pelvis, it is more important to understand the pelvis as a whole, and to appreciate the manner in which it allows the foetal head to pass through during the process of labour. Consideration must therefore be given to the different regions of the pelvis, irrespective of individual bones, joints and ligaments.

THE REGIONS OF THE PELVIS

The Pelvic Brim

It is most important first of all to recognize the structures which comprise the brim of the pelvis. If a finger is placed on the promontory of the sacrum in a model pelvis and is passed around the brim, it will be found to touch the following structures in the order quoted:

i. The promontory of the sacrum.
ii. The wing of the sacrum.
iii. The upper part of the sacro-iliac joint.
iv. The ilio-pectineal line.
v. The ilio-pectineal eminence.
vi. The inner and upper border of the superior ramus of the pubis.
vii. The inner and upper border of the body of the pubis.
viii. The inner and upper border of the symphysis pubis.

The brim of the pelvis, traced in this way on both sides, forms a more or less oval area which divides the pelvis into two portions:

(a) *The False Pelvis,* which lies above the pelvic brim and consists mainly of the iliac fossae. This is of little importance in midwifery.

(b) *The True Pelvis,* which lies below the level of the pelvic brim. This is of great importance, and must be studied in detail.

The True Pelvis

The true pelvis is separated from the false pelvis by the pelvic brim. It consists of three constituent parts:

(a) The inlet or brim of the pelvis.
(b) The cavity of the pelvis.
(c) The outlet of the pelvis.

A. The Inlet or Brim of the Pelvis

The boundaries of this structure are described above. In the normal female gynaecoid pelvis it is approximately oval in shape, the maximum transverse diameter bearing a ratio of 7/6 to the antero-posterior diameter. It is a flat surface, and could be occupied by a flat sheet of paper cut to the appropriate shape. This flat surface is known as the *plane of the brim.*

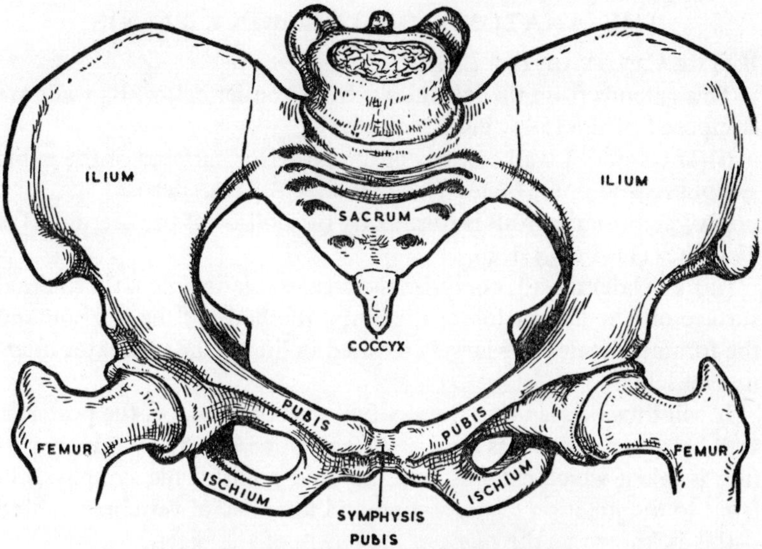

FIGURE 28. View of pelvis from above

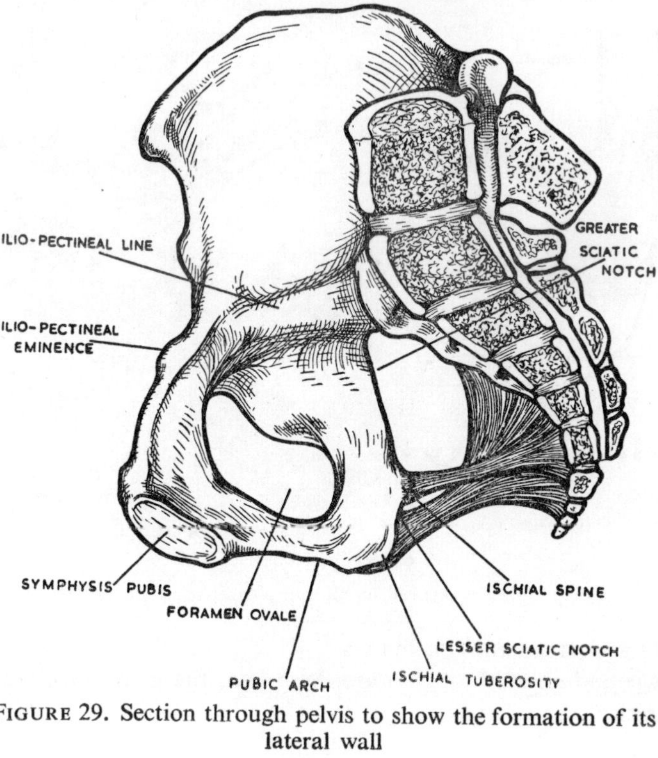

FIGURE 29. Section through pelvis to show the formation of its lateral wall

B. The Cavity of the Pelvis

This extends from the inlet above to the outlet below. Its walls are composed of the following structures:

(i) The anterior wall consists of the posterior surfaces of the pubic symphysis and pubic bones. It is 1½ inches (3·8 cm.) deep.

(ii) The posterior wall is formed by the hollow of the sacrum. It is 4½ inches (11·4 cm.) deep.

(iii) The lateral walls comprise the greater sciatic notch, the internal surface of a small portion of the ilium, the body of the ischium and the foramen ovale. It is largely covered in life by the obturator internus muscle.

It will thus be seen that the cavity is curved in shape, the posterior wall being three times as long as the anterior wall. An imaginary surface is taken which extends from the mid-point of the symphysis in front to the junction of the second and third sacral vertebrae behind —this is known as the *plane of the cavity* of the pelvis.

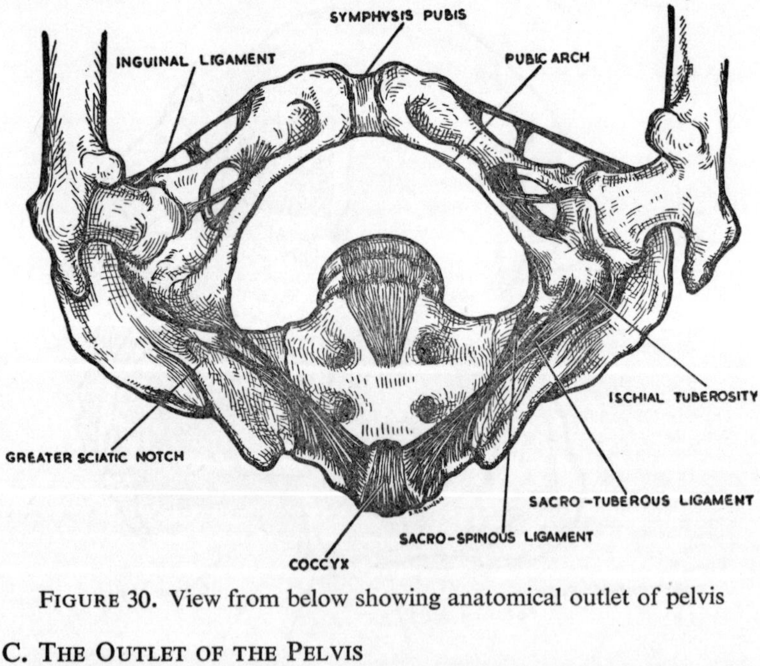

FIGURE 30. View from below showing anatomical outlet of pelvis

C. The Outlet of the Pelvis

Two outlets of the pelvis are described, the anatomical and the obstetrical.

1. *The anatomical outlet.* This is formed by the structures which mark the lower border of the pelvis. Tracing them around the pelvis they are as follows:

i. The lower border of the pubic symphysis.
ii. The pubic arch.
iii. The inner border of the ischial tuberosity.
iv. The sacro-tuberous ligament.
v. The tip of the coccyx.

To the obstetrician and midwife this outlet has certain practical disadvantages. Thus it does not form a flat surface but one which rises and falls as it is traced around the periphery; also its size during

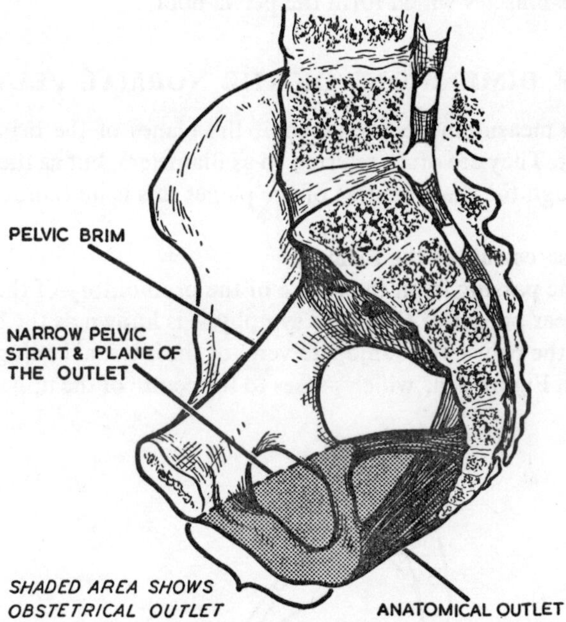

FIGURE 31. The Obstetrical Outlet of the Pelvis

labour is variable, depending upon the range of backward movement of the coccyx that occurs at this time.

2. *The obstetrical outlet.* This is the constricted lower portion of the pelvis and not merely its lower bony border. It is a segment of the pelvis which lies between the anatomical outlet below and an artificial line above. The structures which mark this line are:

(i) The lower border of the pubic symphysis.

(ii) A line passing obliquely across the pubis, foramen ovale and ischium to the ischial spine.

(iii) The sacro-spinous ligament.

(iv) The lower border of the sacrum.

The upper surface of the obstetrical outlet, demarcated by this line, is a flat surface known as the *plane of the outlet*. It is nearly constant in size during labour, being independent of the movements of the coccyx, and is the narrowest part of the pelvis. It is sometimes known as the narrow pelvic strait. The obstetrical outlet is thus a segment of the pelvis, lying between the plane of the outlet (or the narrow pelvic strait) above and the anatomical outlet below, and it is occupied in life by the muscles which form the pelvic floor.

THE DIMENSIONS OF THE NORMAL PELVIS

Certain measurements are taken of the planes of the brim, cavity and outlet. They are often referred to as diameters, but as they do not pass through the exact centres of the planes this is inaccurate.

The Measurements of the Brim

1. A line passing from the centre of the promontory of the sacrum to the upper border of the pubic symphysis is known as the true conjugate of the pelvis, the conjugata vera, or the internal conjugate. The line AB in Figure 31a, which passes to the centre of the upper surface

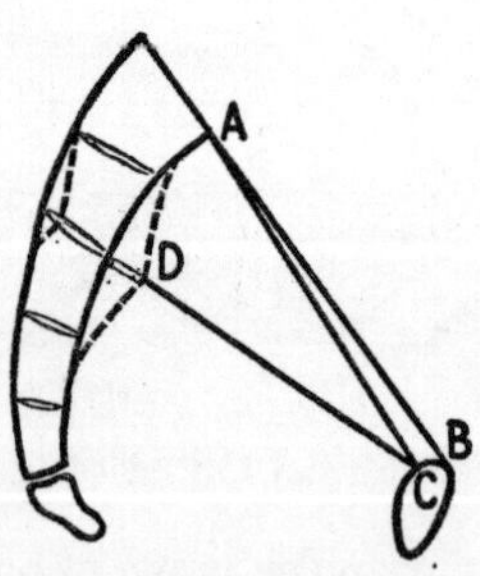

AB anatomical true conjugate
AC obstetrical true conjugate
DC effective true conjugate in cases of false promontory

FIGURE 31a. Types of True Conjugate

of the symphysis, is called the anatomical true conjugate, whereas the line AC which passes to the posterior border of its upper surface, and is the shortest distance between the sacral promontory and the pubic symphysis, is of more value to the obstetrician, and is called the obstetrical true conjugate. It should measure 4½ inches (11·4 cm.) in length.

2. A line passing between the points farthermost apart on the ilio-pectineal lines constitutes the transverse diameter of the pelvic brim. It measures 5¼ inches (13·3 cm.). It cuts the true conjugate in its middle third, the part of the true conjugate lying behind the point of intersection being known as the posterior sagittal diameter of the brim.

3. The oblique diameters pass from the sacro-iliac joints to the

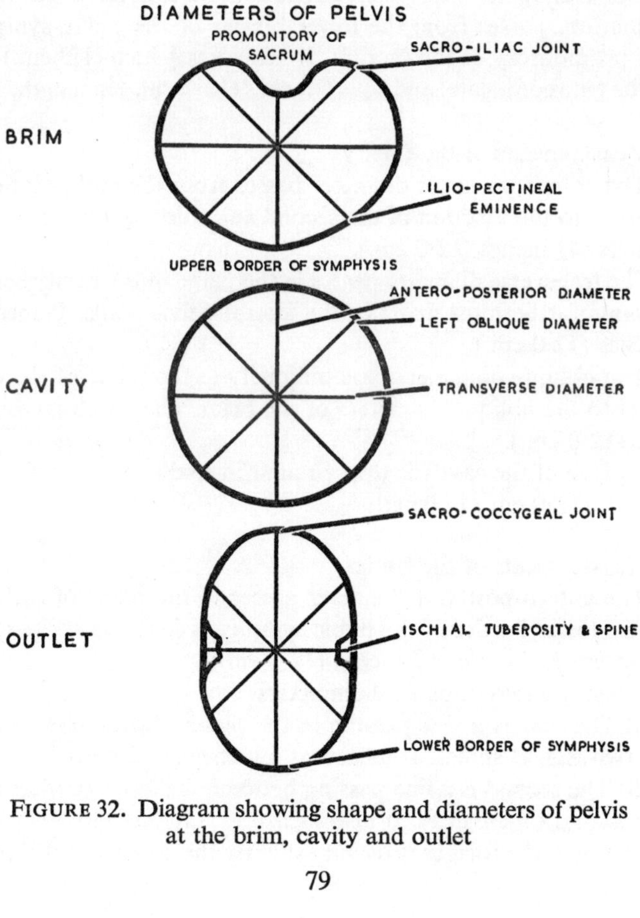

FIGURE 32. Diagram showing shape and diameters of pelvis at the brim, cavity and outlet

opposite ilio-pectineal eminences. The right oblique passes from the right joint, and the left from the left joint. They both measure 4¾ inches (12·0 cm.) in length.

4. Another measurement sometimes described is the sacro-cotyloid diameter. This is a line passing from the promontory of the sacrum to the ilio-pectineal eminence. It measures 3¾ inches (9·5 cm.) on each side.

The inlet is thus an oval structure, which is made heart-shaped by the projecting promontory, with its narrowest diameter running antero-posteriorly and its greatest diameter transversely.

It is impossible to measure the true conjugate directly during life by clinical examination, and it is found indirectly by first measuring the diagonal conjugate. This line, which can be estimated on vaginal examination, passes from the lower border of the pubic symphysis to the promontory of the sacrum. It measures ½ inch (1·3 cm.) more than the true conjugate, and so is 5 inches (12·7 cm.) in length.

The Measurements of the Cavity

1. The antero-posterior diameter passes from the mid-point of the symphysis to the junction of the second and third sacral vertebrae. It measures 4¾ inches (12·0 cm.).

2. The transverse diameter passes in the plane of the cavity between the points farthermost apart in the lateral pelvic walls. It measures 4¾ inches (12·0 cm.).

3. The oblique diameters pass obliquely in the plane of the cavity parallel to the oblique diameters of the brim. They each measure 4¾ inches (12·0 cm.).

The plane of the cavity is thus circular in shape, with all diameters 4¾ inches (12·0 cm.) in length.

The Measurements of the Outlet

1. The antero-posterior diameter passes in the plane of the outlet from the lower border of the pubic symphysis to the lower border of the sacrum. It measures 5 inches (12·7 cm.).

2. There are two transverse diameters:

(i) The first is a line passing in the plane of the outlet between the two ischial spines. It measures 4 inches (10·1 cm.).

(ii) The second is a line passing between the inner borders of the two ischial tuberosities. It also measures 4 inches (10·1 cm.).

Of the two, the former is usually slightly the smaller and therefore

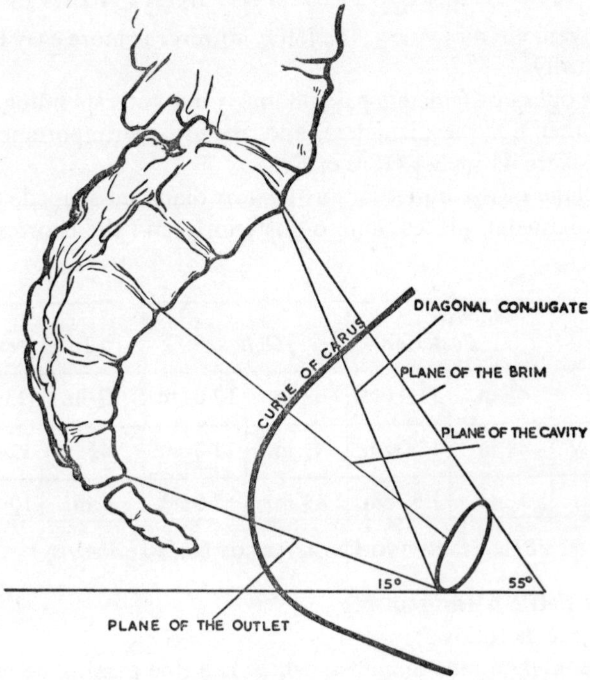

FIGURE 33. Diagram of pelvis showing its three planes and the curve of Carus

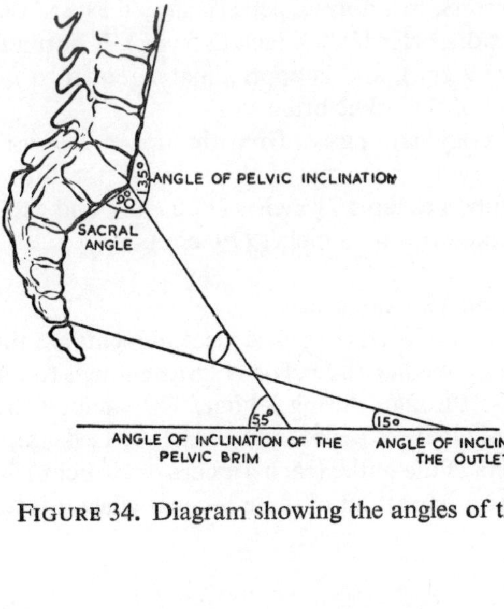

FIGURE 34. Diagram showing the angles of the pelvis

of more value in midwifery; the latter however is more easy to measure clinically.

3. The oblique diameters pass obliquely in a corresponding manner to the other oblique diameters, and are of little importance. They each measure 4¾ inches (12·0 cm.).

The plane of the outlet is thus oval or diamond-shaped, with the longest diameter placed antero-posteriorly and the shortest transversely.

	Antero-Posterior		*Oblique*		*Transverse*	
Brim	4½ in.	11·4 cm.	4¾ in.	12·0 cm.	5¼ in.	13·3 cm.
Cavity	4¾ in.	12·0 cm.	4¾ in.	12·0 cm.	4¾ in.	12·0 cm.
Outlet	5 in.	12·7 cm.	4¾ in.	12·0 cm.	4 in.	10·1 cm.

TABLE SHOWING DIAMETERS OF NORMAL PELVIS

External Pelvic Measurements

These are as follows:

1. The interspinous diameter, which is a line passing between the outer borders of the anterior superior iliac spines. It normally measures 10 inches (25·4 cm.).

2. The intercristal diameter passes between the points farthermost apart on the iliac crests. In a normal pelvis it should exceed the length of the interspinous diameter by one inch (2·5 cm.). It normally measures 11 inches (27·9 cm.), and is approximately equal to twice the transverse diameter of the pelvic brim.

3. The external conjugate passes from the upper anterior border of the pubic symphysis to the tip of the spine of the fifth lumbar vertebra. It normally measures 7½ inches (19·0 cm.), and exceeds the true conjugate of the brim by 3 inches (7·6 cm.).

Significance of Pelvic Measurements

The most important of all these pelvic measurements are the shortest, as they indicate whether the pelvis is large enough to allow the foetal head to pass through during labour. The smallest diameters are thus the true conjugate of the brim (4½ inches or 11·4 cm.) and the transverse diameters of the outlet (each 4 inches or 10·1 cm.). The true conjugate is the most important of these because when it is too short to allow the head to pass, normal delivery is impossible and labour becomes obstructed. When the transverse diameters of the outlet are too short, normal delivery may still be possible if the antero-posterior diameter of the outlet is sufficiently long, for it then allows the head to pass behind the ischial spines rather than between them. Obstructed labour at the outlet occurs only when both the transverse and antero-posterior diameters of the outlet are shortened.

Contraction of the pelvis at the brim is more common than contraction at the outlet.

External measurements are too inaccurate for modern midwifery and their use has now practically fallen into abeyance.

The Axes of the Pelvis

Imaginary lines which pass through the centres of the planes at right angles to them are known as the axes of the pelvis. Those most usually described are:

1. The axis of the brim, which corresponds to an imaginary line passing from the umbilicus to the coccyx.

2. The axis of the outlet, which corresponds to a perpendicular line dropped from the sacral promontory on to the plane of the outlet.

These lines indicate the direction in which the foetus must travel to pass through the plane; hence the foetus passes downwards and backwards to enter the pelvis, and downwards and forwards to emerge from it. This is a result of the inequality in lengths of the anterior and posterior pelvic walls.

3. The pelvic axis is described as an imaginary line which joins the mid-points of successive planes through the pelvis. It marks the direction the foetus moves during birth, passing down the cavity as far as the ischial spines and then curving forwards. It corresponds approximately to a circle described by Carus, which is known as the Curve of Carus.

The Angles of the Pelvis

There are five angles in the pelvis whose importance should be appreciated:

1. *The angle of pelvic inclination* is the angle between the plane of the brim and the anterior surface of the fifth lumbar vertebra. It indicates the angle through which posterior lateral flexion of the head occurs when it becomes engaged with the occiput in a lateral position, and it should not exceed 135°.

2. *The sacral angle* is the angle between the plane of the brim and the anterior surface of the first sacral vertebra. It usually measures 90°. It indicates the dimensions of the cavity relative to the size of the brim, for if the angle is less than 90° the cavity is smaller than the brim, whilst if it exceeds 90° the cavity is larger.

3. *The inclination of the brim* is the angle the plane of the brim makes with the horizontal, the patient being in the erect attitude. It is usually about 55°. Thus in the standing position the upper border of the symphysis is in the same vertical plane as the anterior superior iliac spines, and in the same horizontal plane as the coccyx.

4. *The inclination of the outlet* is the angle the upper border of the obstetrical outlet makes with the horizontal. It amounts to 15°, and is of little significance.

5. *The pubic angle* is the angle between the two ischio-pubic rami which form the pubic arch. In the normal female gynaecoid pelvis this measures about 90°.

Variations in Pelvic Shape

The normal female pelvis which has been described above occurs in approximately 50 per cent of Anglo-Saxon women. It is known as a gynaecoid pelvis, in contrast to the pelves of the remaining 50 per cent of women, where certain variations are to be found. These differences are best seen on X-ray examination when they may be classified into the following types:

1. *The android brim.* (23 per cent of patients.)

A brim of this type possesses certain characteristics of the male pelvis, being wedge-shaped with the apex of the wedge in front. Posteriorly a straight sacrum and a flattened promontory form the hind-pelvis, laterally the ilio-pectineal lines are relatively straight, and anteriorly they meet at an angle to form a narrow fore-pelvis. The maximum transverse diameter crosses the true conjugate in its posterior third close to the sacrum, resulting in a shortened posterior sagittal segment. Although the diameters of the brim may be equal to those of the gynaecoid shape, yet the space available for the passage of the foetus is considerably reduced.

Sometimes the android brim is associated with a characteristic cavity and outlet, when the whole pelvis may be said to be an android pelvis. In this event, the sacrum tends to be relatively straight throughout its whole length, the bones are large and the ischial spines prominent. The greater sciatic notches are narrow and the sacro-spinous ligaments short, whilst the pubic angle measures less than a right angle. All the outlet measurements may be reduced and the pelvis then constitutes one type of funnel pelvis.

2. *The anthropoid brim.* (24 per cent of patients.)

This type of brim has features similar to that of the anthropoid apes, and is characteristically long and narrow. It results from a reduction in the size of the maximum transverse diameter so that its normal 7/6 ratio to the true conjugate is diminished. Sometimes in fact the transverse diameter becomes equal to or smaller than the conjugate. It still, however, crosses the conjugate in its middle third, whilst the hind and fore-pelves are average in size or a little narrow.

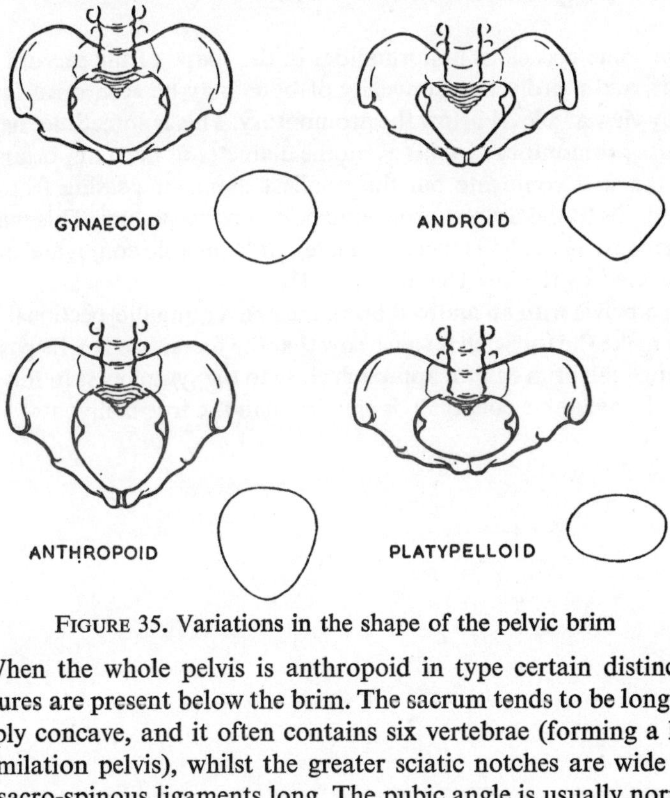

FIGURE 35. Variations in the shape of the pelvic brim

When the whole pelvis is anthropoid in type certain distinctive features are present below the brim. The sacrum tends to be long and deeply concave, and it often contains six vertebrae (forming a high assimilation pelvis), whilst the greater sciatic notches are wide and the sacro-spinous ligaments long. The pubic angle is usually normal.

3. *The platypelloid brim.* (3 per cent of patients.)

This type of brim is characteristically flattened, with the true conjugate reduced in size and the maximum transverse diameter elongated, so that there is at least an inch (2·5 cm.) difference between them.

When the platypelloid features involve the whole pelvis, reduced antero-posterior diameters and increased transverse diameters are present in the cavity and outlet, whilst the pubic angle may be wider than normal.

Many pelves, however, cannot be classified into these four types because they bear features characteristic of more than one group. When this occurs the hind and fore-pelves are allocated separately to the type to which they belong, and the brim is called andro-gynaecoid, or gynaeco-android, etc., as the case may be. The shape of the hind-pelvis is always stated first.

On some occasions abnormalities in the shape of the sacrum may occur, and a projecting convexity of bone may be seen on a lateral X-ray view at a level below the promontory. This is sometimes named a 'false promontory'. In this event the diameter of most importance is not the true conjugate but the smallest diameter passing from the symphysis to the nearest projecting point on the sacrum. This may be referred to as the 'effective conjugate', or 'available conjugate' and is illustrated by the line DC in Figure 31a.

In a pelvis with an android brim, the converging ilio-pectineal lines may make the fore-pelvis so narrow that the foetal head on its passage through the brim cannot approach close to the symphysis. In this case also the available conjugate is smaller than the true conjugate.

CHAPTER 4

The Physiology of Menstruation

A full understanding of the phenomenon of menstruation requires knowledge firstly of the ovarian changes associated with ovulation, and secondly of the uterine changes preceding the actual blood flow. Ovulation is best understood by first considering the changes which affect the ovary in different age groups.

THE OVARY AT DIFFERENT AGES

1. In the Female Foetus and Young Girl

The ovary in a young female foetus is a solid organ, conforming to the anatomy already described in Chapter 1. On section the cortex of each ovary is found to contain about 200,000 primordial follicles. These consist of a large central cell, containing a prominent nucleus, which is enveloped by a single layer of small flattened cells. Each of these central cells is an ovum which is capable in later life of becoming matured and fertilized and then developing into a baby; it can be seen from this that the female is lavishly endowed by nature with reproductive elements. The primordial follicles are separated from each other by the ovarian stroma—a connective tissue containing spindle cells—and are enclosed within the tunica albuginea and germinal epithelium.

When the foetus is 36 weeks old, changes begin in some of the primordial follicles and persist throughout infancy and early girlhood. These changes consist of an increase in the number of capsular cells, which become in consequence many layers thick around the ovum. This is followed by the appearance of fluid between the cells, known as the liquor folliculi. In this way some of the primordial follicles become converted into small cystic follicles, which are known as Graafian follicles.

2. During Sexual Life

The Graafian follicles remain quite small until the girl reaches puberty, when she is about thirteen to fourteen years of age. After this they become much larger and some gradually attain a diameter of 8 to 12 mm.

Structure of a Graafian Follicle

The structures which comprise a Graafian follicle from within outwards are as follows:

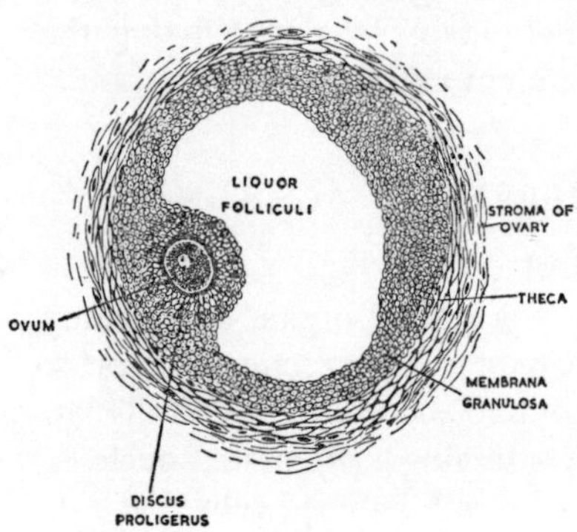

FIGURE 36. A Graafian follicle

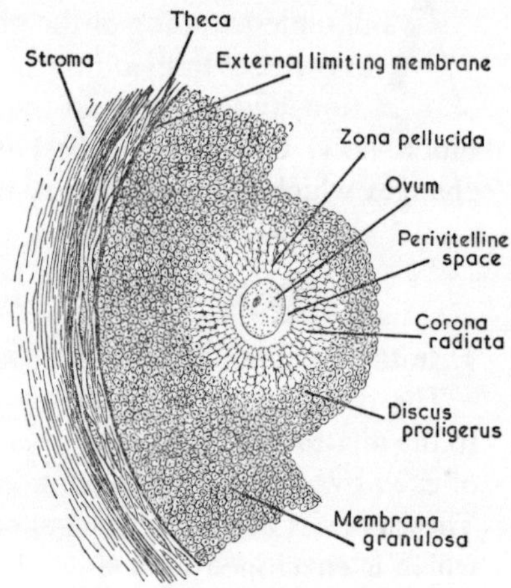

FIGURE 36a. An enlarged view of the ovum and discus proligerus

(i) A large central cell, about $\frac{1}{160}$ inch or 0·15 mm. in diameter, which is known as the ovum. It contains a large nucleus, with prominent nucleoli, and has many fat globules and particles scattered throughout its cytoplasm.

(ii) Immediately outside the ovum is a very narrow space, the perivitelline space.

(iii) Surrounding the ovum and the perivitelline space is a large clump of cells attached at one pole to the lining of the follicle. These cells are known as granulosa cells, and the clump they form around the ovum is called the discus proligerus.

The cells of the discus next to the perivitelline space are arranged in such a manner that they appear to radiate from the ovum—this formation is called the corona radiata. These coronal cells contain amorphous material which forms a translucent membrane, the zona pellucida, lying immediately adjacent to the perivitelline space.

(iv) The follicle itself is lined with granulosa cells similar to those of the discus proligerus; these constitute the membrana granulosa or the zona granulosa. Scattered between the granulosa cells, especially near the discus proligerus prior to ovulation, are small globules of clear fluid surrounded by a ring of granulosa cells—these are known as Call-Exner bodies.

(v) The follicle is filled with fluid—the liquor folliculi—which lies between the zona granulosa and the discus proligerus. It is probably formed by the granulosa cells.

(vi) Externally the zona granulosa cells rest upon a basement membrane which encloses the whole follicle. This is called the membrana limitans externa or external limiting membrane.

(vii) Outside the follicle the stroma of the ovary is compressed to form a capsule, which is known as the theca. This is usually formed of two parts, an inner vascular layer known as the theca interna or theca vasculosa, and an outer layer named the theca externa or theca fibrosa. These layers are more marked in lower animals than in human beings.

After ovulation has occurred the ovary also contains corpora lutea which are described later.

3. The Post-Menopausal Ovary

After the menopause, which usually occurs between 46 and 50 years of age, no follicles or corpora lutea are to be found in the cortex, which then consists only of fibrous tissue. The ovary is thus reduced to an atrophic shrunken body, with a scarred irregular surface.

THE MECHANISM OF OVULATION

The sexual phase of a woman's life begins at puberty, when she is about thirteen to fourteen years of age, the appearance of the first menstrual period being called the menarche, and extends until menstruation ceases at the menopause, usually when she is aged forty-six to fifty. During this time one Graafian follicle each month outstrips its fellows and develops in size until it is about 16 mm. in diameter. It then protrudes from the surface of the ovary, with the discus proligerus and the contained ovum lying in its most projecting part. As it enlarges, the ovarian capsule is increasingly stretched, until it becomes so thin that it breaks. The follicle thus ruptures, and the liquor folliculi, the discus proligerus and the ovum are cast out into the peritoneal cavity. This process is known as ovulation.

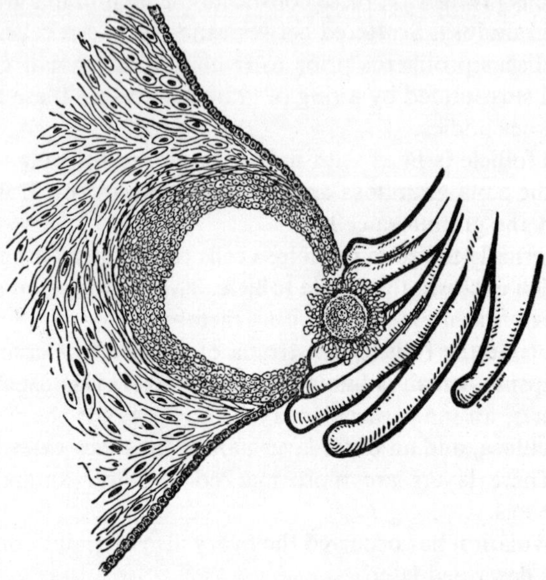

FIGURE 37. Drawing of the actual process of ovulation

At the time of ovulation the fimbrial end of the Fallopian tube lies in close apposition to the follicle, and as the ovum with its mantle of cells is cast out, it is wafted by peritoneal currents set up by the ciliated cells of the tube into its lumen, along which it travels towards the uterus.

Ovulation takes place each month in alternate ovaries, so that each individual ovary ovulates at two-monthly intervals. During a woman's life, therefore, ovulation occurs some 400 times, so that very few of the original 400,000 primordial follicles reach full development.

Ovulation is sometimes accompanied by pelvic pain, which is known as Mittelschmerz. This may be due to the stretching of the ovarian capsule, to slight bleeding into the peritoneal cavity, or to peristalsis in the Fallopian tube occurring at this time.

The Corpus Luteum of Menstruation

After ovulation the empty follicle becomes collapsed, and a little bleeding sometimes occurs into its cavity. It no longer remains circular in shape, but becomes wavy in outline, or crenated, owing to the crumpling of its collapsed walls. The cells of the membrana granulosa, which are left behind after ovulation, now begin to enlarge and proliferate, so that after a few days a small solid body, about 1 cm. in diameter, wavy in outline and greyish-yellow in colour, is formed at the site of the previous Graafian follicle. This is the corpus luteum, the enlarged granulosa cells now being known as granulosa lutein cells. The cells of the theca interna also proliferate and invade the corpus luteum between its convolutions—they are called paralutein cells.

The corpus luteum grows for 14 days and becomes yellow in colour, after which time hyaline material is deposited between its cells and it begins to atrophy. The granulosa lutein cells become vacuolated and undergo degeneration, the colour of the corpus luteum gradually changing from yellow to white. During the succeeding weeks the cells of the corpus luteum disappear, and after nine months it has become converted into a small hyaline nodule, known as a corpus albicans.

Hormonal Control of Ovulation

The growth and ripening of the Graafian follicles are under hormonal control, the regulating hormone being derived from the basophil cells of the anterior lobe of the pituitary gland, which is situated within the skull on the under surface of the brain. This hormone belongs to the class of pituitary gonadotrophins, and is known as follicle-stimulating-hormone or FSH. It is carried in the bloodstream from the pituitary to the ovary where it causes a follicle to grow and enlarge, and at the same time stimulates the cells of the zona granulosa and the theca interna to produce another hormone called oestradiol.

When the amount of this hormone reaches a certain level, the further production of FSH is stopped and a second pituitary gonadotrophic hormone, luteinizing hormone or LH, is produced. When the falling FSH and the rising LH reach a certain ratio, they cause the follicle to rupture and ovulation to occur.

After ovulation the development and growth of the corpus luteum are brought about by LH. This persists for 14 days, after which its secretion by the pituitary stops, FSH reappears, and the cycle is repeated.

Some authorities believe that another pituitary gonadotrophic hormone known as luteotrophin or LTH (which is identical with prolactin that stimulates the production of milk in the breasts during the puerperium) is responsible for the development of the corpus luteum, but this is doubtful.

Thus, for two weeks preceding ovulation, the ovary is under the influence of FSH, and for the two subsequent weeks it is under that of LH. The ultimate degeneration of the corpus luteum is brought about by the withdrawal of its trophic secretion LH, and its substitution by FSH which follows causes fresh growth in another Graafian follicle in the opposite ovary. In this way, the cycle continues (unless interrupted by pregnancy or disease or hormone therapy) throughout the sexual phase of a woman's life.

The anterior lobe of the pituitary is linked to the neighbouring part of the brain, known as the hypothalamus, by a special system of veins, the pituitary portal system. The production of gonadotrophic hormones from the anterior pituitary is regulated by the hypothalamus through these portal veins. As the hypothalamus is connected by nerve tracts with the higher cortical centres, it can be appreciated that emotional factors may influence the occurrence of ovulation and interfere with menstruation.

Hormonal Secretion by the Ovary

The Graafian follicles and corpora lutea are not only under the hormonal influence of pituitary gonadotrophins, but they also secrete hormones on their own account.

1. During the development of the Graafian follicle, oestradiol is secreted by the cells of the zona granulosa and the theca interna. It is stored in the liquor folliculi and later passes round the body producing the effects described below. After ovulation it is secreted in lesser amounts by the corpus luteum and is also formed in the cortex of the suprarenal glands. It is metabolized in the liver and is excreted mainly in the urine in the form of oestriol and oestrone and some eight other related compounds. These substances are known as oestrogens, and are responsible for the secondary sex characteristics which appear in the young girl at the time of puberty, and for some of the changes that occur during the menstrual cycle and pregnancy.

The chief effects induced by oestrogens are:

(i) The production of the typical feminine shape of the waist and hips, with soft skin and smooth gentle curves, resulting from the deposition of fat in the subcutaneous tissues which occurs at puberty.

(ii) The growth of the breasts and nipples, the former being chiefly due to the development of the duct system.

(iii) The development of the adult vulva and vagina. The squamous epithelium of the vagina, which is thin in childhood, becomes thicker, and the superficial cells become cornified after puberty. These cells, when they desquamate, encourage the proliferation of Döderlein's bacilli by virtue of the glycogen they contain, and the increased lactic acid they produce brings about the marked acidity of the adult vagina.

(iv) The growth of the uterus at puberty, the development of the uterine muscle, and proliferative changes in the endometrium during the menstrual cycle, as described below. The cervical glands also increase in size and produce a greater quantity of mucus, which on drying crystallizes into a pattern resembling fern leaves when seen under a microscope. This result of oestrogenic stimulus constitutes what is known as the 'fern test'.

(v) The inhibition of FSH and prolactin from the anterior pituitary, but not LH. The changes in the levels of FSH and LH are responsible for ovulation, as previously described.

(vi) The retention of water and electrolytes in the body tissues.

(vii) During pregnancy, the growth of the uterine muscle, and the ducts of the breasts. It is the continuous high level of oestrogens during this time which, by means of pituitary inhibition, suppresses ovulation and lactation in pregnancy.

2. The cells of the corpus luteum, under the influence of LH (or LTH), produce another hormone known as progesterone, and a small quantity of oestrogens. The changes produced in the body by progesterone are very important, but they are chiefly manifested during pregnancy, when it is produced in large quantities. Apart from pregnancy its chief function is to produce endometrial changes as part of the menstrual cycle.

The main effects of progesterone are:

(i) The production of secretory changes in the endometrium prior to menstruation.

(ii) To cause slight tingling in the breasts before the onset of menstruation.

(iii) To cause a slight rise in the body temperature of about half a degree.

(iv) During pregnancy:

(a) The formation of the decidua in the uterus, which enables the fertilized ovum to become embedded.

(b) The relaxation of the tone of smooth muscle throughout the body.

(c) The enlargement of the breasts, by growth of the milk-forming alveoli.

(d) The retention of water and electrolytes in the body tissues in association with oestrogens.

Atretic Follicles

A word should be said about the majority of the primordial follicles which do not undergo full development into Graafian follicles. Many of these simply disappear, but others become partially developed and then reach a standstill. Hyaline material is then laid down under the membrana limitans externa, forming what is known as the glass membrane. The constituent cells of the follicle gradually disappear and become replaced by the glass membrane. These follicles are known as atretic follicles.

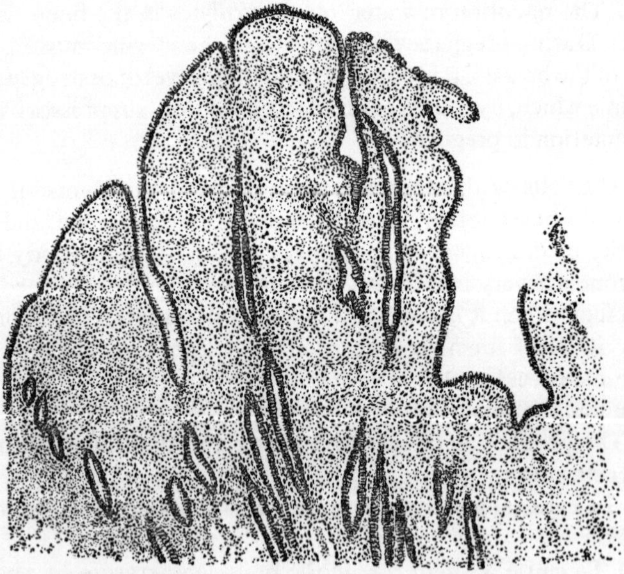

FIGURE 38. Proliferative endometrium, showing straight tubular glands under the influence of oestrogens. (*Low-power magnification*)

THE PHYSIOLOGY OF MENSTRUATION

UTERINE CHANGES ASSOCIATED WITH MENSTRUATION

The uterine changes which relate to menstruation occur in the corporeal endometrium as a result of its stimulation by the ovarian hormones, the oestrogens and progesterone. These take the forms of the proliferative phase when the endometrium is under the influence of oestrogens, the secretory phase when it is under the influence of oestrogens and progesterone together, and finally the actual phase of menstruation itself.

1. The Proliferative Phase

This begins at the end of a menstrual period, when the actual loss of menstrual blood ceases, and lasts thereafter for about ten days. During this time a Graafian follicle is ripening in an ovary, and it is the oestrogens from the granulosa cells and theca interna of the follicle which are responsible for the changes which take place.

These consist of the repair of the denuded endometrium, whose superficial layer has been cast off during menstruation, by growth from the unchanged deeper layer, and its subsequent hypertrophy until it is about 3·5 mm. thick.

The structure of this proliferated endometrium is as follows:

(i) A basal layer about 1 mm. in thickness, which lies on the myometrium. It consists of a loose connective tissue containing spindle cells, lymphocytes collected into lymphatic nodes, and blood-vessels. It contains the tips or extremities of the tubular uterine glands, some of which terminate in this layer, whilst others invade the myometrium for a short distance. This zone remains unchanged during all the phases of menstruation.

(ii) A superficial layer, 2·5 mm. in thickness, composed of loose connective tissues containing tubular glands, spindle cells, blood-vessels and lymphatics. This is known as the functional layer. The tubular glands are narrow, of uniform width, and pass straight from the surface down to the basal layer.

(iii) The epithelium which covers the functional layer is cuboidal and ciliated in places. It is this epithelium which dips down into the endometrium to form the tubular glands.

2. The Secretory Phase

After the proliferative phase of the endometrium has been in exis-

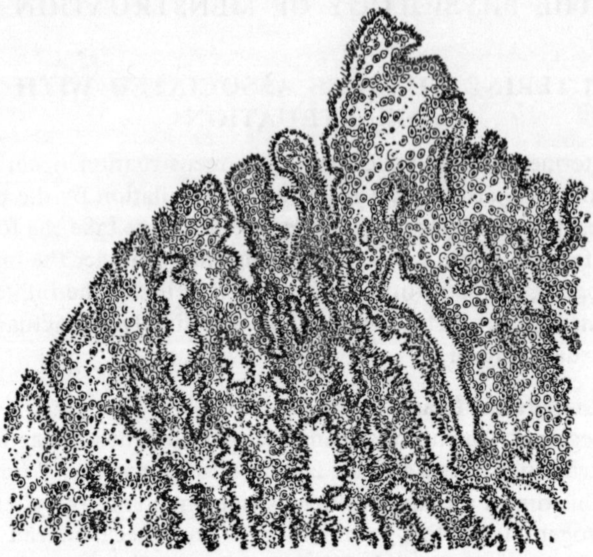

FIGURE 39. Secretory endometrium, showing corkscrew glands under the influence of progesterone. (*Low-power magnification*)

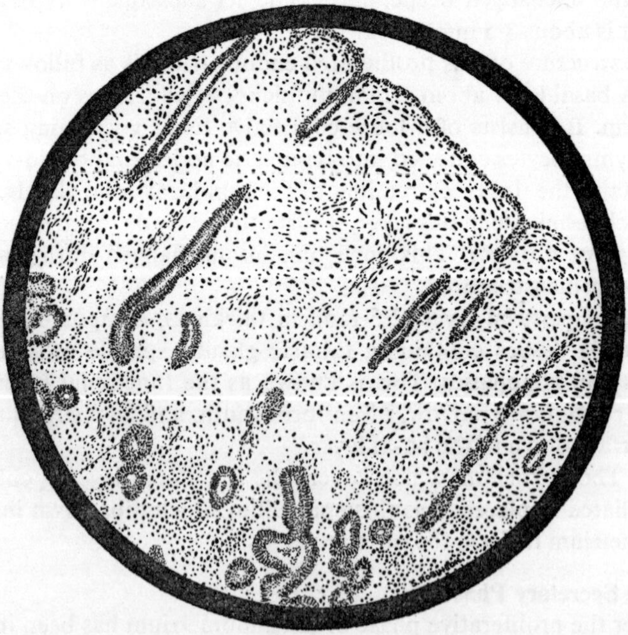

FIGURE 40. Drawing of the compact layer of the functional endometrium (*High-power magnification*)

tence for about ten days, ovulation occurs in the ovary and the corpus luteum is formed. The progesterone from the corpus luteum produces the following changes in the endometrium, which constitute the secretory phase which lasts for 14 days:

(i) The basal layer remains unchanged.

(ii) The functional layer increases in thickness up to 3·5 mm. The glands become widened and dilated, and further increase in length so that they become corkscrew-shaped; their cells are filled with secretion which passes into the lumen of the glands. The spindle cells become enlarged and are clumped together mainly in the superficial zone of the endometrium. The functional layer after the twenty-first day of the cycle comes to consist of two zones:

(a) A superficial compact zone filled with swollen stromal cells.

(b) A deeper spongy layer composed of dilated glands lying in a loose connective tissue framework. Towards the end of the fourteen days the endometrium becomes increasingly vascular and congested.

(iii) The surface epithelium remains unchanged.

3. The Menstrual Phase

After fourteen days of life the corpus luteum degenerates, the supply of oestrogens and progesterone is cut off from the endometrium and in consequence the functional layer dies. It is the disintegration of the functional layer of the endometrium, with consequent bleeding, which constitutes the actual menstrual flow. The arteries in the endometrium are spiral in form; immediately before menstruation begins, short segments of these vessels go into intermittent spasm. At the same time anastomotic channels open up between the arterioles and veins in the superficial layers of the endometrium, so that the blood is shunted from the arterioles directly into the veins, and the circulation through the capillaries of the superficial layers is brought to a standstill. Deprived of its circulation, the functional part of the endometrium undergoes necrosis and sloughs off, being subsequently expelled from the uterus by muscular contractions. It is this tissue, accompanied by bleeding from disrupted blood-vessels, which actually forms the menstrual flow. This usually continues for about four days, the total amount of blood lost amounting to some 50 to 100 grammes, containing 25 mg. of iron, whilst the presence of special ferments prevents the blood from clotting. The ovum in a degenerated state is also passed during this time.

At the end of this phase a new endometrium is reconstituted from the unchanged basal layer containing the terminal deep portions of the tubular glands, as already described.

RELATION OF MENSTRUATION TO OVULATION

It will be understood that normal menstruation is completely dependent upon the hormonal changes associated with ovulation, which are themselves related to changes in the anterior lobe of the pituitary gland. Ovulation occurs fourteen days before the onset of the next menstrual period, and as the ovum only remains capable of being fertilized for 24–48 hours thereafter, women are thus in their most fertile state about fourteen days before the next menstrual period is expected.

The menstrual rhythm may be tabulated thus:

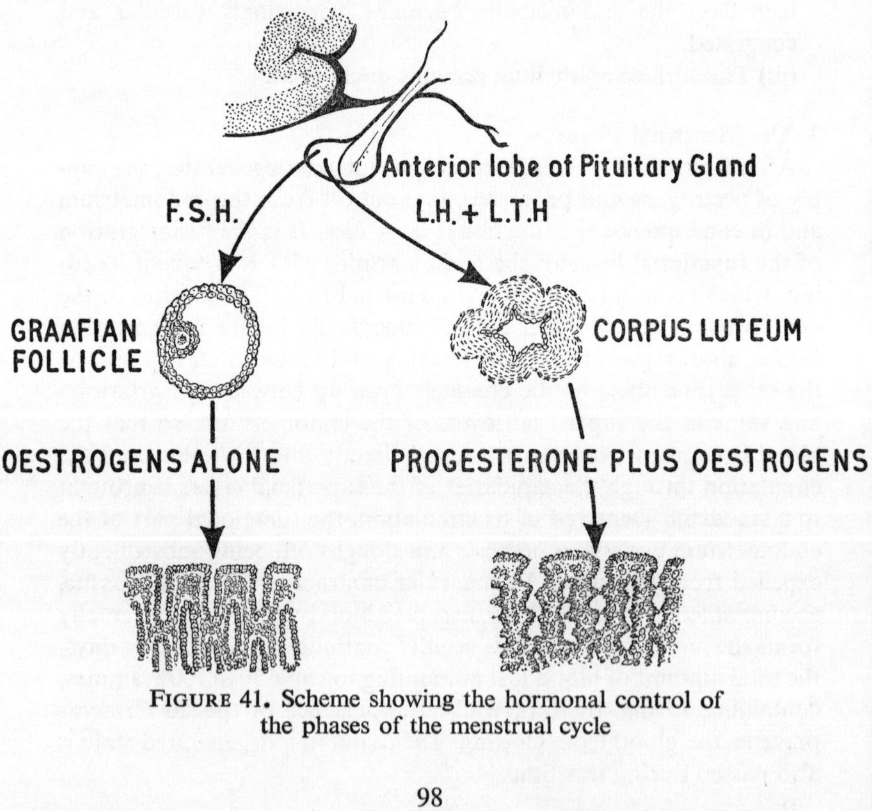

FIGURE 41. Scheme showing the hormonal control of the phases of the menstrual cycle

	Duration in Days
1. Following menstruation there is growth of a follicle; production of oestrogens; proliferative changes in the endometrium	10
2. Ovulation	–
3. Growth of a corpus luteum; progesterone production with a small amount of oestrogens; secretory changes in the endometrium	14
4. Degeneration of corpus luteum and menstruation	4
(*see* FIG. 42) Total	28

This sequence occurs every four weeks under normal circumstances, and in the absence of pregnancy, from the time of puberty until the menopause. Individual variations in these figures are, however, quite common. Thus menstruation may last from 2 to 7 days, and may occur at intervals of 3 to 6 weeks and still be quite normal. Ovulation, however, in these cases always occurs about fourteen days before the onset of the next period, so that the length of the secretory phase is approximately constant, whilst the proliferative phase varies with the duration of the cycle.

Significance of Menstruation

The whole of the menstrual process is a preparation for pregnancy, because the fertilized ovum needs a rich and vascular membrane in which to grow and develop. The secretory endometrium, formed after ovulation, is such a membrane, and its whole purpose is to provide a suitable nidus for the development of the fertilized ovum. If such an ovum is not produced, the endometrium is cast off when it grows stale after fourteen days and a new one is substituted. Thus for the children which a woman bears, 400 suitable endometria are provided during the course of her lifetime; this is typically in keeping with the opulence of natural processes, where austerity is unknown. To produce her children, approximately 400 ova leave the ovaries, and each has an especial secretory endometrium prepared for its possible reception; to provide 400 ova, 400,000 primordial follicles originally exist. Truly nature spares nothing when it makes preparations for the propagation of the race!

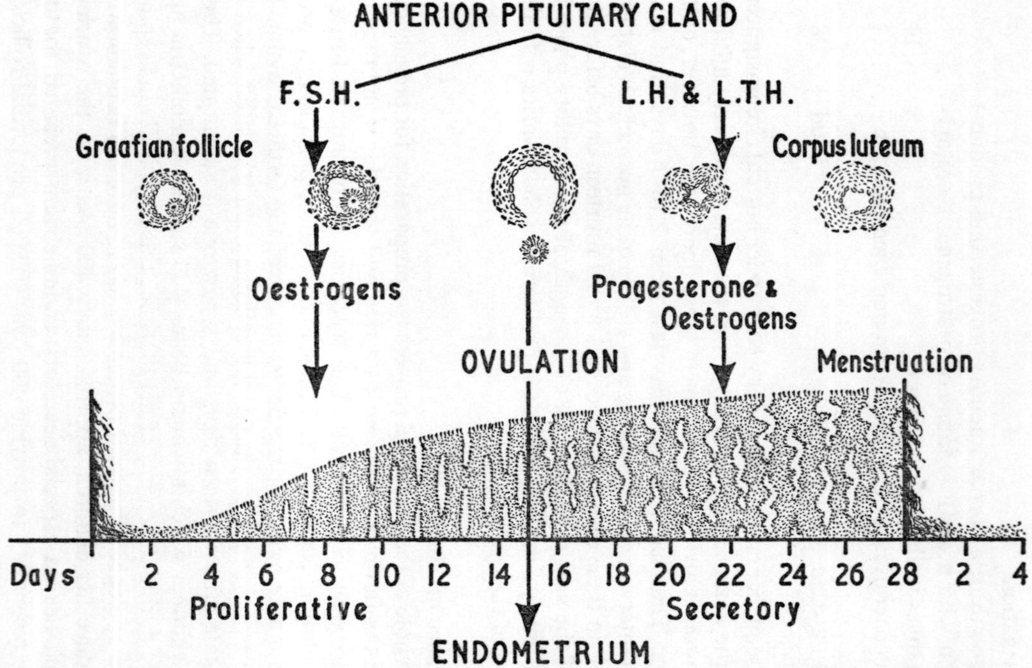

FIGURE 42. Scheme showing relation of ovarian and endometrial changes to the menstrual cycle

CHAPTER 5

The Development of the Fertilized Ovum During Early Pregnancy

Having considered the changes associated with ovulation and menstruation in the non-pregnant woman, attention must now be given to the sequence of events which ensues when pregnancy supervenes.

MATURATION OF THE OVUM

Prior to the act of ovulation, certain changes take place in the ovum (whilst it is still within the Graafian follicle) which constitute what is known as the maturation of the ovum. This consists essentially of a division of the ovum, whereby the number of chromosomes in the nucleus is reduced from 46, the normal number in human beings, to 23.

Normally when every cell in the body divides, the nucleus splits up into 46 small threads of nuclear material known as chromosomes. These become divided longitudinally during normal cell division so that each daughter cell still contains the full number of 46 chromosomes. Exceptions to this rule occur during maturation of the ovum and during development of the spermatozoa from the primary spermatocytes in the male testes, when the number of chromosomes is halved, so that the human reproductive cells each contain only 23.

Each chromosome is composed of clumps of nuclear material, in the same way that a chain is made up of links. These are known as genes, about 2,000 being present in each chromosome. It is these genes which impart to the individual his specific physical, mental and moral characteristics which together make up his appearance, intellectual powers and behaviour.

When maturation of the ovum takes place the two resultant cells, each containing 23 chromosomes, are very unequal in size. One cell is still called the ovum and exactly resembles the ovum in size before maturation; the second cell is very small and consists merely of nuclear material surrounded by a small amount of cytoplasm. This cell is known as the first polar body. It may be said, then, that the ovum undergoes maturation prior to ovulation by casting off the first polar body. Further details of this process are described in Appendix III, page 194.

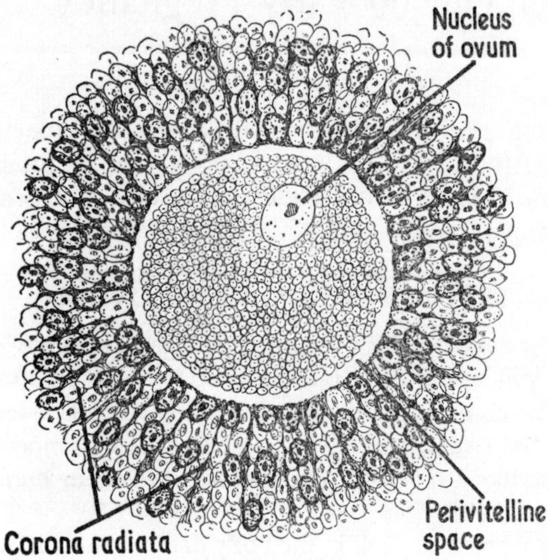

FIGURE 43. Drawing of an ovum surrounded by the discus proligerus

FERTILIZATION OF THE OVUM

After ovulation the ovum, surrounded by its mantle of cells, the corona radiata, is received into the Fallopian tube. It passes slowly down the tube towards the uterus, moving along as a result of waves of peristalsis in the walls of the tube, aided by currents set up by the ciliary action of the lining cells. During this time the ovum receives food partly from the cells of the corona, and partly from secretions of the cells in the mucosa of the Fallopian tube.

When sexual intercourse occurs semen containing a large number of spermatozoa is deposited in the upper vagina. The liberality of natural processes is again here demonstrated, because the actual number of spermatozoa ejaculated at this time is about 300,000,000, of which only one is necessary to effect fertilization.

The human spermatozoon is a small structure 1/420 inch (60μ) in length, shaped rather like a tadpole, and comprising a head, neck, middle piece and tail. The head is shaped like a pointed oval, and is covered by a hemispherical cap known as the head-cap or acrosome. It contains 23 chromosomes and is largely composed of deoxyribonucleic acid (DNA) (See Appendix III, p. 194). Next to the head is a small constricted neck which contains the centriole of the cell. The middle piece consists of an axial bundle of fibrils surrounded by a coiled sheath of mitochondria, the fibrils being continued down the long tail. It is by lashing movements of the tail that the spermatozoon is able to travel along the female genital tract, covering its own length in 3 seconds, a speed corresponding to 3 inches (7·5 cm.) an hour. These movements of the tail are controlled by the mitochondria, which use a special form of sugar known as fructose in the semen as a source of energy.

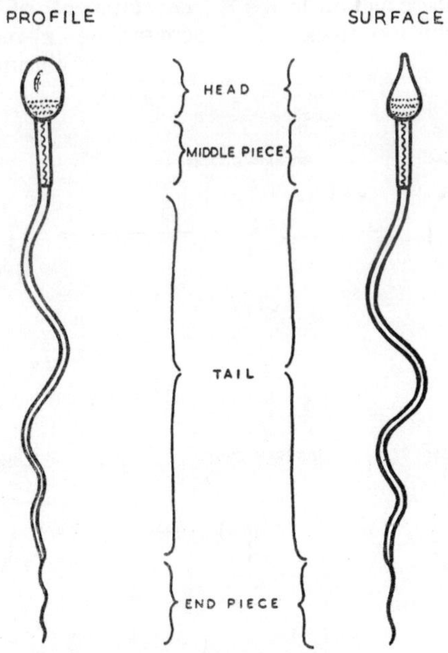

FIGURE 44. Spermatozoa (*High-power magnification*)

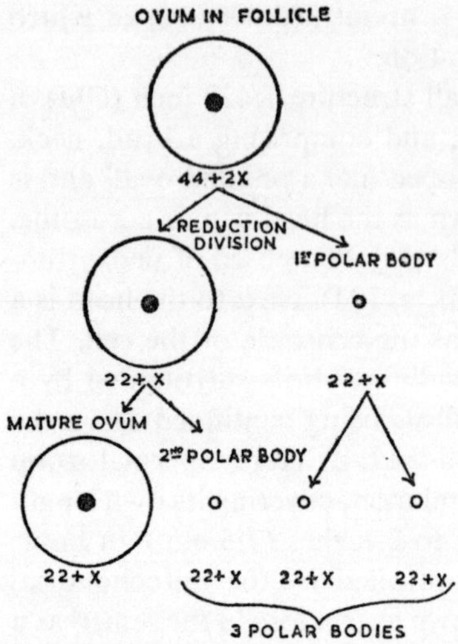

FIGURE 45. Scheme showing maturation of ovum, with reduction in the number of chromosomes

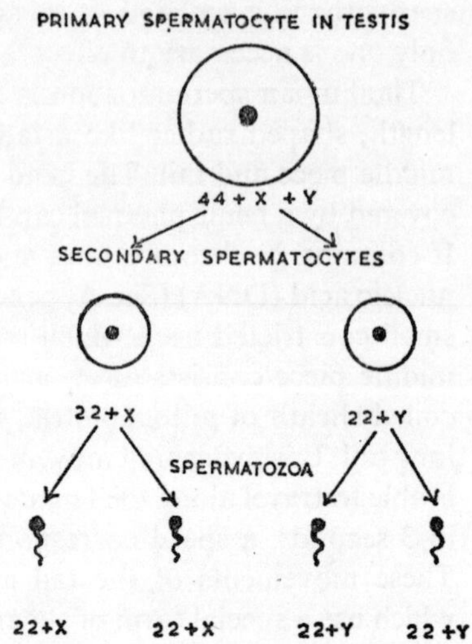

FIGURE 46. Scheme showing similar development of spermatozoa also containing a reduced number of chromosomes

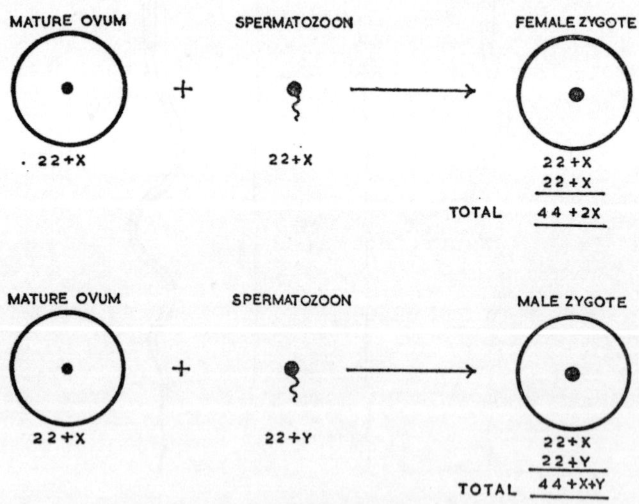

FIGURE 47. Scheme illustrating the formation of male and female zygotes

FERTILIZED OVUM DURING EARLY PREGNANCY

After the act of intercourse many of the spermatozoa are killed by the lactic acid present in the vaginal fluid. Spermatozoa live best in an alkaline medium, and this is provided by the excretion of alkaline mucus from the cervical glands. Thus after a few hours many of the spermatozoa are killed, but those that have reached the haven of a drop of cervical mucus survive; they are then able to reach the external os, to work their way up the cervical canal, and to pass through the uterine cavity into the Fallopian tubes.

The spermatozoa which enter the tubes are able to travel against the direction of peristalsis and ciliary flow by virtue of the propelling action of their tails. Those which have entered the tube containing the ovum reach it in the outer third of the Fallopian tube. The ovum remains capable of fertilization only for 24–48 hours after ovulation, during which time it occupies this part of the tube.

Many spermatozoa arrive at the discus proligerus which they then have to penetrate in order to reach the ovum. They are able to do this by means of an enzyme which they carry known as hyaluronidase. This breaks down the cementing substance holding the cells of the discus together without actually destroying them—the spermatozoa are thus able to pass between the cells to reach the ovum. One spermatozoon then unites with it by entering into its substance. As soon as this occurs the cell membrane becomes impenetrable and no further spermatozoa are able to effect a union. This entry of a spermatozoon into the ovum constitutes the essential feature of fertilization.

After the entry the head of the spermatozoon forms a mass of nuclear material, containing 23 chromosomes, which is known as the male pronucleus; the middle piece and tail drop off and are merged into the cytoplasm of the ovum. The other unwanted spermatozoa throughout the female genital tract atrophy and disappear.

Following the entry of the spermatozoon, further changes take place in the nucleus of the ovum, whereby a second polar body is formed and cast off. There is no further reduction in the number of chromosomes at this division, so that the now mature ovum and the second polar body each contain 23 chromosomes. The first polar body may also divide at this time so that 3 polar bodies may be present alongside the ovum; these however serve no known function, but degenerate and disappear. The nucleus of the mature ovum is now known as the female pronucleus. The cell thus contains a male pronucleus of 23 chromosomes and a female pronucleus of 23 chromosomes; fusion of these 2 structures then occurs and a cell containing 46 chromosomes results. This is described in greater detail in Appendix III, page 194.

This cell is a new individual and is known as a zygote. The qualities it possesses, derived from its genes, come half from its mother and half from its father; although its nutrition is derived solely from its mother for many months, yet it is a true blend of the qualities of its two parents.

At the time of fusion of the pronuclei the sex of the new individual is decided. This is because the sex of the individual is a function of its constituent chromosomes. Thus the human cell of 46 chromosomes is made up of 44 ordinary chromosomes plus two sex chromosomes of different kinds, one known as X and the other as Y. Female cells contain 44 plus 2 X chromosomes, and male cells 44 plus X plus Y. After the reduction division all ova contain 22 plus X chromosomes, whilst spermatozoa are of two kinds—some contain 22 plus X, whilst others contain 22 plus Y. The sex of the zygote depends upon the kind of spermatozoon which effects fertilization; if this is done by a 22 plus X type, the zygote will contain 44 plus 2 X chromosomes and will develop into a female; if a 22 plus Y type, it will contain 44 plus X plus Y, and will consequently become male. The sex of the offspring, in human beings, is thus solely dependent upon the father.

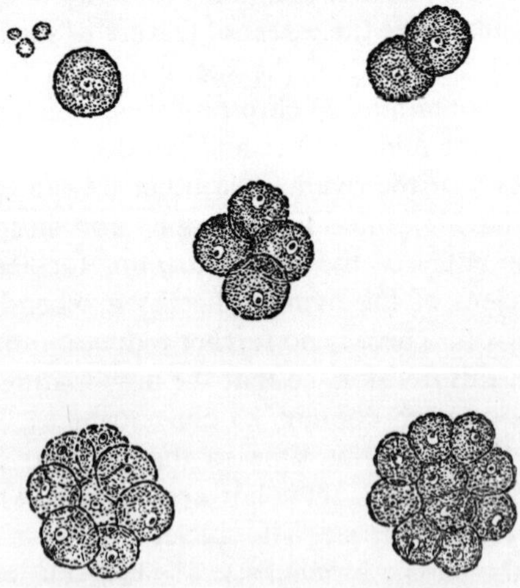

FIGURE 48. Diagram of the fertilized ovum undergoing segmentation

SEGMENTATION OF THE OVUM

At the time of fertilization the ovum is still within the zona pellucida and corona radiata lying in the outer third of the Fallopian tube. After fertilization the zygote travels along the tube and reaches the uterus in about four days, being nourished by secretions from the goblet cells in the epithelium lining the tube and by degenerating cells of the discus proligerus. During this time the zygote divides into two cells, then into four and eight, and so on. This process is known as the segmentation of the fertilized ovum, and the mass of cells produced, about ½ mm. in diameter, is known as the morula. The zona pellucida serves to bind the cells together and to prevent their adherence to the walls of the tube, but it disappears by the time the cavity of the uterus is reached.

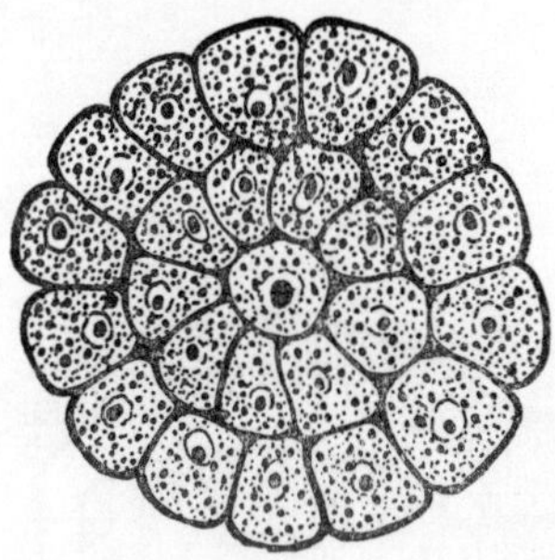

FIGURE 49. Diagram of a morula

During this journey some fluid appears between the cells of the morula, and a small cystic structure 2mm. in diameter, known as the blastocyst, is formed. It is at this stage that the fertilized ovum enters the uterine cavity, 4 days after fertilization, and 5 or 6 days after ovulation. The capsule of the blastocyst is composed of a layer of cells known as the trophoblast, whilst at one pole is collected a small mass of cells which is called the inner cell mass. As the blastocyst lies in the uterine cavity the cells of the trophoblast lie adjacent to the surface of the secretory endometrium; from the time of the seventh day after fertilization two simultaneous events begin to occur, namely the formation of the decidua and the embedding of the ovum.

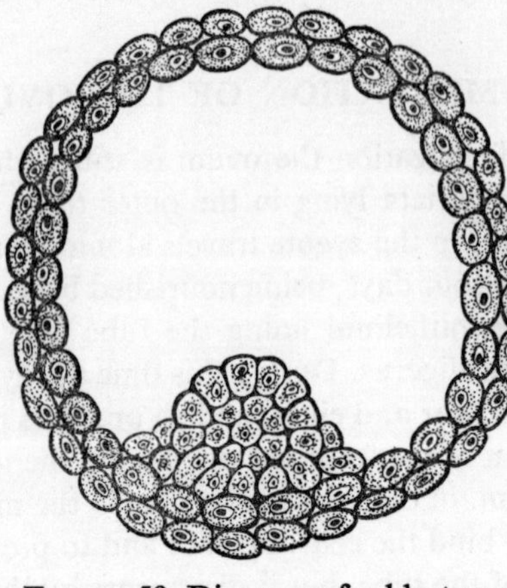

FIGURE 50. Diagram of a blastocyst

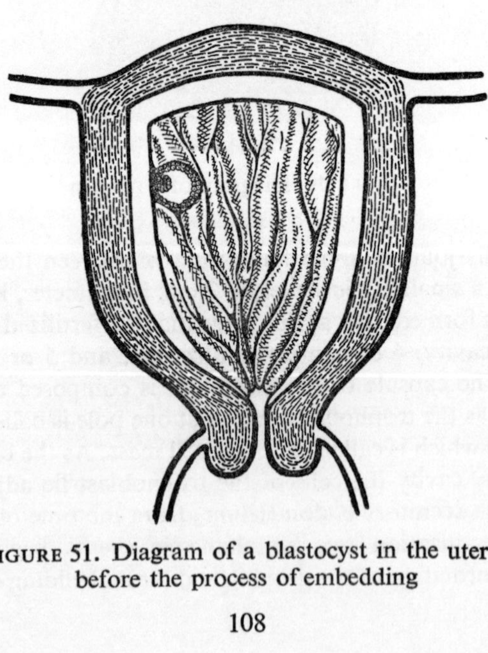

FIGURE 51. Diagram of a blastocyst in the uterus before the process of embedding

THE FORMATION OF THE DECIDUA

As the embedding of the ovum (which will presently be described) is in progress, changes occur in the secretory endometrium which result in its becoming transformed into the decidua. These changes are as follows:

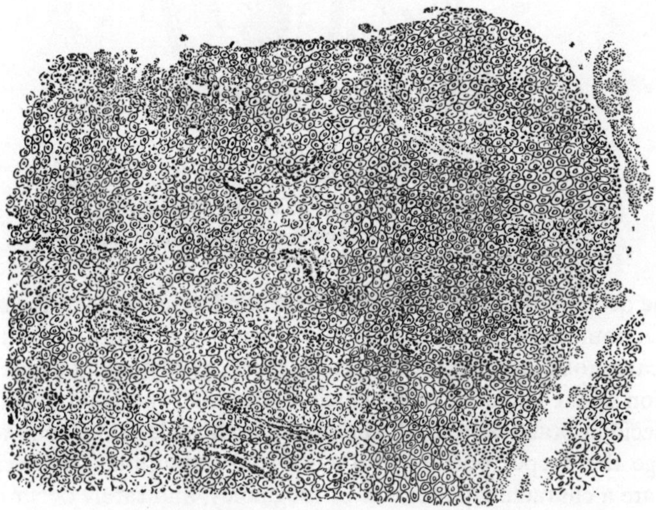

FIGURE 52. Drawing of the compact layer of the decidua (*High-power magnification*)

1. The endometrium hypertrophies, reaching 6 to 8 mm. in thickness.
2. The stroma becomes increasingly vascular and oedematous.
3. The stroma cells swell and enlarge with the result that they become closely packed together in the superficial part of the functional layer. They now form what is known as the compact layer. These new cells, which are called decidual cells, are polygonal in shape as a result of the mutual pressure they exert upon each other.
4. The tubular glands become more tortuous and dilated in their deeper parts, and their lumina are packed with secretion. This increased dilatation below the compact part of the functional layer produces a spongy cavernous appearance; it is known as the cavernous layer.
5. The basal layer remains unchanged.

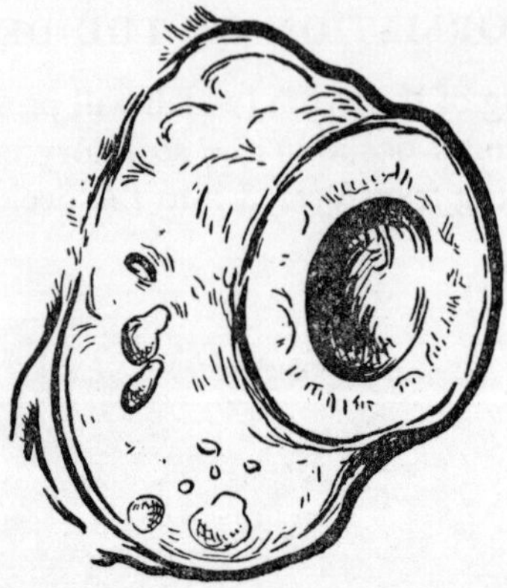

FIGURE 53. Section of ovary showing cystic corpus luteum of pregnancy

The decidua thus is thicker, more rich and vascular than the secretory endometrium. The division of the functional layer into compact and cavernous layers is much more marked, partly owing to the production of the decidual cells, which render the superficial portion of the decidua practically solid, and partly to the enlarged glands which change the deeper portion into a net-like formation. The decidual cells are a characteristic feature of pregnancy, and rarely occur apart from it.

This development of the decidua results from an increased output of progesterone from the corpus luteum. Accordingly it is found that the corpus luteum in the presence of pregnancy does not degenerate in the usual way at the fourteenth day after ovulation, but instead continues to grow and develop. In fact, it increases in size up to the twelfth week of pregnancy, when it becomes cystic and occupies one third of the entire ovary. It is this greatly enlarged corpus luteum of pregnancy which provides the progesterone responsible for the building up of the decidua; also as degeneration does not occur, there is no death of the endometrium and no menstruation; hence this increased growth of the corpus luteum and production of progesterone are responsible for the amenorrhoea associated with pregnancy.

The stimulus which makes the corpus luteum develop in the presence of an embedding ovum is hormonal. A gonadotrophic hormone is produced from the cells of the trophoblast as they invade the lining of the uterus. This hormone, known as chorionic gonadotrophin or the APL principle (anterior-pituitary-like), is absorbed into the maternal blood from the invading trophoblast, and is carried to the ovary. Here it augments the action of LH from the anterior pituitary, with the result that increased growth and development of the corpus luteum ensue.

It is this hormone, chorionic gonadotrophin, which, excreted into the urine, is used as a basis for animal pregnancy tests which are employed to diagnose the existence of pregnancy, for it is only found when trophoblast cells, and therefore pregnancy, are present.

THE EMBEDDING OF THE OVUM

As the blastocyst rests on the surface of the endometrium where it

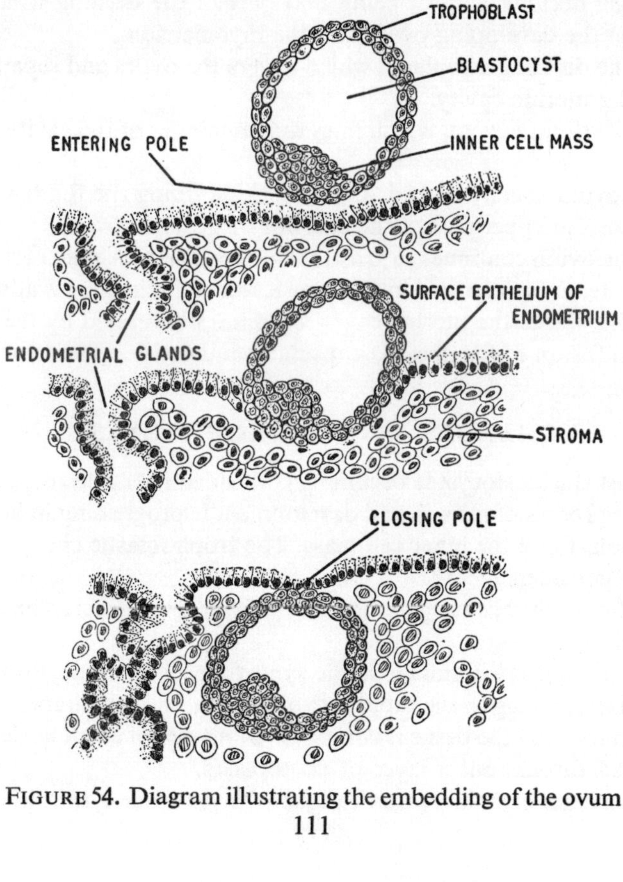

FIGURE 54. Diagram illustrating the embedding of the ovum

is nourished by secretions from the uterine glands, the trophoblast cells excrete ferments which digest the endometrial cells and so form a small scooped-out depression in which the blastocyst rests. This begins about the seventh day after fertilization. The digestive process continues and the blastocyst sinks deeper and deeper into what is now becoming the decidua, the deepest cells constituting the entering pole, to which the inner cell mass is attached. Finally the whole blastocyst is received into the decidua, the last portion to enter being the closing pole, and the superficial part of the decidua closes over the blastocyst, its site of entry being marked by a small fibrin plug.

At this stage the blastocyst forms a small nodule lying in the decidual lining of the uterus; it bulges progressively more into the uterine cavity as it continues to enlarge. The decidua thus becomes divided into three parts:

1. The decidua basalis, being that part of the decidua which lies between the developing ovum and the myometrium.
2. The decidua capsularis, which covers the ovum and separates it from the uterine cavity.
3. The decidua vera, which lines the remainder of the cavity of the uterus.

The ovum usually embeds in the decidua lining the fundus of the uterus or the upper part of the anterior or posterior walls.

As the ovum continues to grow, the uterus enlarges at an even more rapid rate, as is described in Chapter 8. When pregnancy is advanced to twelve weeks the uterine cavity becomes obliterated by the meeting and fusion of the decidua capsularis and the decidua vera.

CHANGES IN THE TROPHOBLAST

Whilst the blastocyst is becoming embedded in the decidua, a continuous process of growth and development is progressing in both the trophoblast and the inner cell mass. The trophoblastic changes must first be considered.

As the trophoblast cells proliferate they become differentiated into three layers:

1. An outer layer known as the syncytium or the syncytiotrophoblast. Here, owing to the rapid rate of growth, the cell boundaries are not formed, and the tissue is composed of masses of small nuclei lying scattered throughout a layer of protoplasm.
2. An inner layer known as Langhans' layer or the cytotrophoblast.

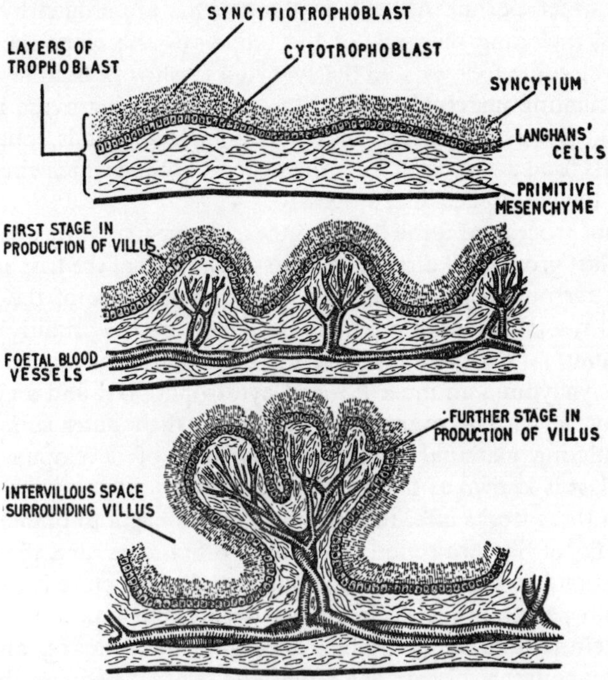

FIGURE 55. Three stages in the formation of villi from the trophoblast

This is composed of single cells with complete cell membranes, known as Langhans' cells, which lie beneath the syncytium.

3. Below the cytotrophoblast lies a layer of loose connective tissue, known as primitive mesenchyme; this is continuous with similar tissue in the inner cell mass, the point where they join being known as the body stalk.

The next changes occur in the outer syncytial layer. Vacuoles appear in this tissue, and as it thickens and increases in size these run together and form a network of little tunnels, as it were, throughout the syncytium. These spaces are known as the chorio-decidual spaces. Thus as the syncytiotrophoblast grows it invades the surrounding decidua, in the form of a network of protoplasmic meshes enveloping the entire ovum.

Digestive ferments are being continuously excreted by the trophoblast during this time, and are responsible for the invasion of the decidua which occurs. All cells in the decidua are eroded by these ferments, including the walls of the blood-vessels; when these are affected bleeding follows, and the syncytial meshwork becomes filled with circulating maternal blood. Thus the developing ovum is first nourished by the secretions of the endometrial glands, but later obtains its food and oxygen from the maternal blood which circulates through the chorio-decidual spaces.

As the process of growth continues, finger-like projections of trophoblast grow in all directions from the surface of the trophoblast into the surrounding decidua, so that the appearance of the ovum comes to resemble that of a porcupine. These are the primitive villi; they contain all the three layers of the trophoblast, having an outer layer of syncytium, an inner layer of cytotrophoblast and a core of mesenchyme, and are everywhere bathed on their outer surface by the circulating maternal blood. At this stage of development the trophoblast is known as the primitive chorion.

About three weeks after fertilization the villi begin to branch, and a single finger-like projection develops two branches, and then four and eight and so on, until a branching tree-like structure is formed. These villi penetrate the decidua very deeply, but however complicated their pattern, they contain the same three layers, and are bathed by maternal blood. The blood-filled spaces between the villi are now known as the intervillous spaces.

At this time a new system of blood-vessels becomes formed in the mesenchymal cores of the villi. The vessels in each branch of the villus join together until fairly large vessels reach its base; here the vessels from adjacent villi unite and form larger vessels which pass in the primitive chorion towards the body stalk and inner cell mass. These form part of the foetal system of blood-vessels. It can thus be understood that food products and oxygen, derived from the maternal blood, pass through the walls of the villi into the foetal blood-vessels, which carry them through the body stalk into the inner cell mass where the foetus is developing.

During the third month of pregnancy some of the villi continue to proliferate whilst others atrophy. Those villi which have invaded the decidua basalis develop a very intricate complicated arborescent pattern, and form what is called the chorion frondosum. The villi in the decidua capsularis become smaller as the decidua stretches, and finally about the twelfth week of pregnancy they disappear, leaving behind a smooth layer of chorion known as the chorion laeve.

During the remaining six months of pregnancy the chorion frondosum develops into the foetal part of the placenta, and the chorion laeve becomes the chorion. Thus it will be understood that the placenta and chorion are both derived from the primitive chorion, which itself is a derivative of the trophoblast.

The villi which form the placenta are of two types:

1. Nutritive villi. These lie free in the maternal blood spaces and are concerned with nutritive processes.

2. Anchoring villi. These are attached by cellular growth at their tips to the deeper layers of the decidua, and therefore in addition to their nutritive function they stabilize the placenta through their attachment to the decidua.

Stability is also achieved by decidual septa which pass into the placenta between clumps of villi and around its edge.

Under normal circumstances the villi do not invade the basal unchanged layer of decidua or the muscle of the uterine wall. Such penetration is stopped by a layer of fibrinoid material which is present in the deeper part of the functional layer of the decidua—this is known as the layer of Nitabuch.

CHANGES IN THE INNER CELL MASS

Whilst the trophoblast is changing into the nutritional organ of the embryo, the inner cell mass is developing into the foetus, and their point of junction, the body stalk, is elongated to become the umbilical cord.

The first change which occurs in the inner cell mass is the appearance within it of two small cavities, each lined with cubical epithelium. These are the amniotic cavity, lined with ectodermal cells (which form the amnion), and the yolk sac, lined with endodermal cells. Between these cavities lie other cells known as mesodermal cells. The remaining cells of the inner cell mass are formed of primitive mesenchyme. Thus in the region where the two cavities come closest together are situated ectoderm, endoderm and mesoderm cells. These are all formative cells from which the entire body is built up—thus all the cells necessary for the formation of the embryo are here present, and this zone between the cavities is therefore called the embryonic plate.

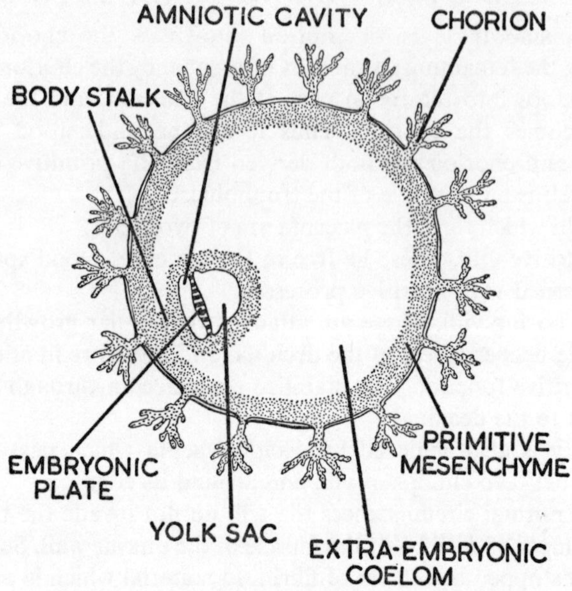

FIGURE 56. Diagram showing early changes in blastocyst

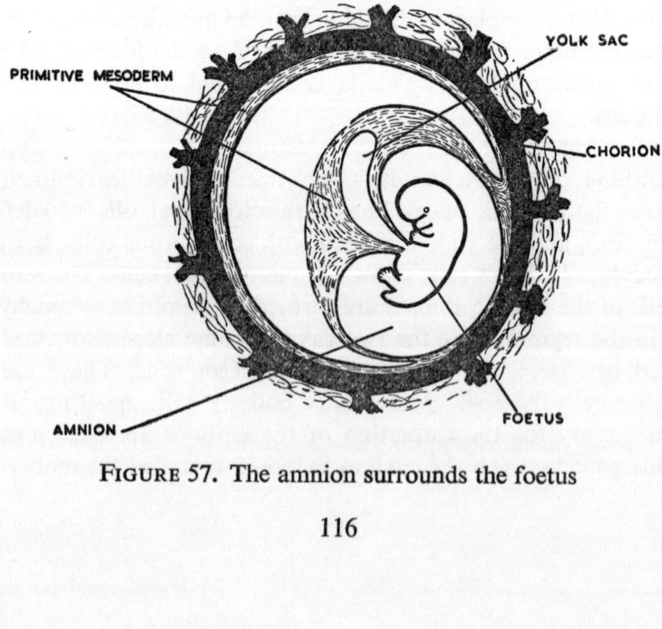

FIGURE 57. The amnion surrounds the foetus

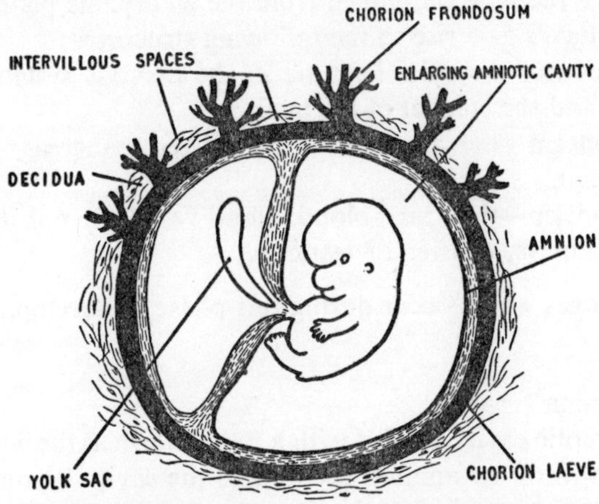

FIGURE 58. The amnion undergoing expansion to line the inside of the trophoblast

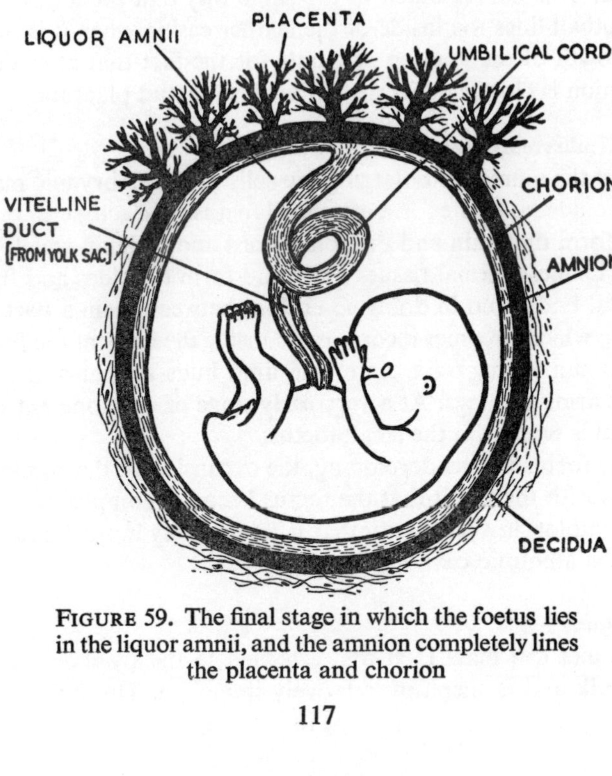

FIGURE 59. The final stage in which the foetus lies in the liquor amnii, and the amnion completely lines the placenta and chorion

When the foetus is developed from the embryonic plate, the three formative layers give rise to the following structures:

1. Ectoderm—the skin, hair, nails, the nervous system, the lens of the eye and the enamel of the teeth.

2. Endoderm—the alimentary tract, liver, pancreas, lungs and thyroid gland.

3. Mesoderm—the heart, blood, blood-vessels, lymphatics, bones, muscles, kidneys, ovaries or testicles.

The changes which occur during this phase of development are as follows:

1. The Amnion

The amniotic cavity is filled with a fluid known as the liquor amnii. Rapid growth of the amnion occurs and the cavity becomes greatly enlarged, so much so in fact that it comes to fill the entire blastocyst. As a result of this expansion the amnion comes to line the inside of the trophoblast, or, as it has by now become, the chorion and placenta. This occurs much in the same way that the inner bladder of a football lines the inside of the leather casing when it is inflated. This growth of the amnion accounts for the fact that after delivery the amnion is closely adherent to the chorion and placenta.

2. The Embryonic Plate

Whilst the amnion is enlarging the cells of the embryonic plate become moulded into the form of a small foetus. The ectoderm proliferates to form the brain and the spinal cord and the skin which covers them. The mesodermal tissues grow and form the sides and front of the foetal body, and in doing so enclose between them a part of the yolk sac, which becomes incorporated inside the body of the foetus to form its alimentary tract. Later the limb buds appear and develop into the arms and legs. At a very early stage of development quite a large tail is present in the small foetus.

As the foetus is thus developing, the expansion of the amnion is in progress with the result that the foetus becomes completely enclosed by the amnion in such a way that it floats freely in the liquor amnii inside the amniotic cavity.

3. The Body Stalk

The inner cell mass is at first attached to the trophoblast at the body stalk and is therefore relatively immobile. Through the body stalk the primitive mesenchyme lining the trophoblast becomes continuous with that in the inner cell mass.

While the expansion of the amnion and the growth of the foetus are in progress, the body stalk becomes greatly elongated and forms the umbilical cord, thereby allowing the foetus to become freely mobile within the liquor. The blood-vessels which run in the body stalk from the trophoblast to the embryonic plate become converted into the umbilical arteries and vein, which pass in the umbilical cord from the placenta to the foetus.

As the expanding amnion encloses the foetus within it, it also surrounds the umbilical cord and fuses with it in such a way that the cells covering the cord and the amnion become continuous with each other.

4. The Yolk Sac

It has already been described how part of the yolk sac becomes enclosed by the growing body of the foetus to form its alimentary tract. The remainder of the yolk sac is caught up in the body stalk and becomes incorporated into the umbilical cord. It can be found after delivery as a small vestigial structure inside the cord which is known as the vitelline duct. Abnormalities of this process give rise to Meckel's diverticulum of the gut, which rarely may extend through the umbilicus into the proximal part of the cord.

The net result of these changes is to produce a mobile foetus, immersed in the liquor amnii, attached to the placenta by its umbilical cord, and surrounded by two sets of membranes, the inner amnion and the outer chorion.

CHAPTER 6

The Physiology of the Foetus and its Appendages During Pregnancy

THE GROWTH OF THE FOETUS

The formation of the embryo from the embryonic plate takes place between the third and eighth weeks of pregnancy. From this time until the end of pregnancy steady growth in the foetus continues, until at term a full-time foetus, weighing about 7 lb. (3,200 grammes) and measuring 20 inches (50·8 cm.) in length is produced. The increase in size of the foetus throughout pregnancy may be seen from the following table:

Weeks of Pregnancy	*Crown to Heel Length of Foetus*		*Weight of Foetus*	
4	—		—	
8	1¼ inches	3·1 cm.	1/30 oz.	0.9 grammes
12	3¼ ,,	8·2 ,,	½ ,,	14·2 ,,
16	6¼ ,,	15·8 ,,	3½ ,,	100 ,,
20	10 ,,	25·4 ,,	8 ,,	227 ,,
24	12 ,,	30·4 ,,	1½ lb.	680 ,,
28	14 ,,	35·6 ,,	2¼ ,,	1,140 ,,
32	16 ,,	40·5 ,,	3½ ,,	1,600 ,,
36	18 ,,	45·7 ,,	5 ,,	2,270 ,,
40	20 ,,	50·8 ,,	7 ,,	3,200 ,,

This table shows that the rate of growth of the foetus is much greater during early pregnancy than it is during the later months, for its length is approximately doubled during each of the early months, whilst during the second half of pregnancy its monthly increase is about 2 inches (5·1 cm.). Its weight increases similarly, although a rapid gain occurs during the last few months due to the deposition of fat in the subcutaneous tissues at this time.

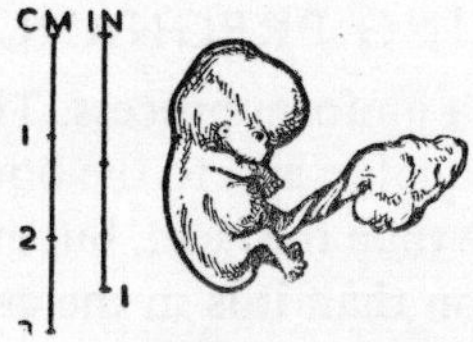

FIGURE 60. A small foetus aged 6 weeks

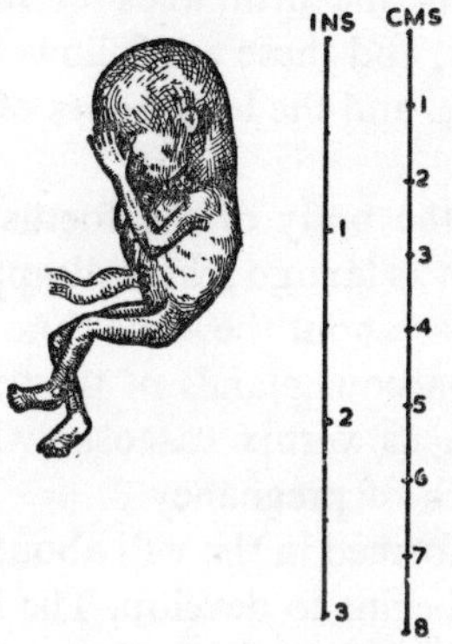

FIGURE 61. A foetus aged 10 weeks

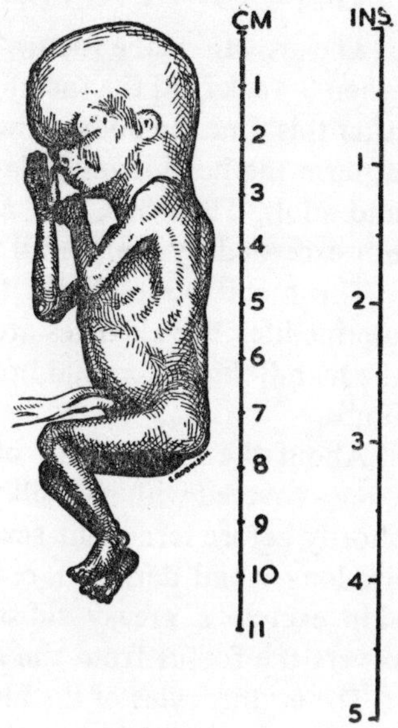

FIGURE 62. A foetus aged 14 weeks

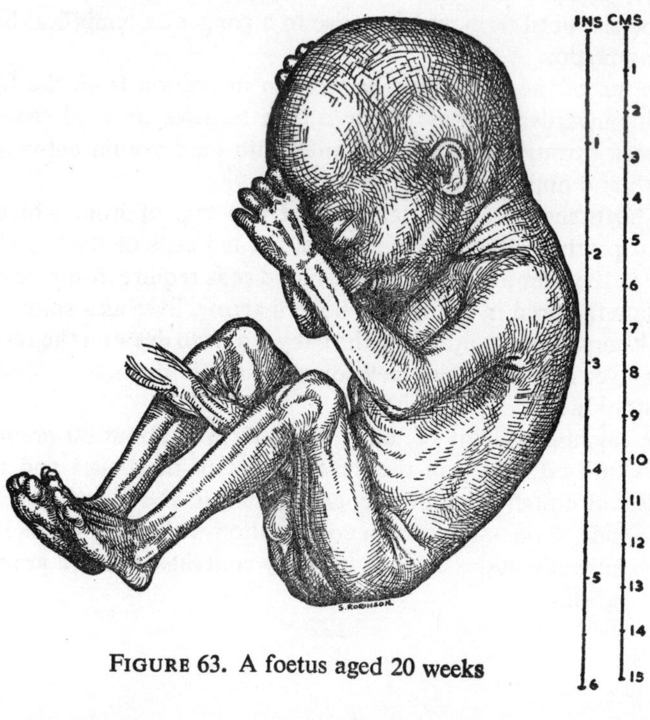

FIGURE 63. A foetus aged 20 weeks

The growth of the foetus, however, is not a uniform process. Thus when 8 weeks old the foetal head is almost equal in size to the body; after this time the body grows relatively more than the head, but even at term the head is much larger in proportion than it is in the child and adult. The arms, too, at term are longer than the legs, and are not exceeded by them until the child is about two years old.

The foetal bones begin to ossify about the fifth week of intra-uterine life. The clavicles are ossified first, and these are followed by the mandible, the cranial bones, vertebrae, and the long bones of the limbs.

About the fifth month of pregnancy the body of the foetus becomes covered with pale silky hairs known as lanugo; these disappear shortly before term. The scalp hairs appear about the same time and are longer and darker in colour. The sebaceous glands of the foetal skin excrete a greasy substance, known as vernix caseosa, which covers the foetus from the seventh month of pregnancy.

The erythrocytes of the blood are first formed in the villi about the third week, at which time the heart also begins to develop. The liver is a large organ during foetal life, filling the upper half of the abdomen; because of this the gut is extruded through the umbilicus into the proximal part of the cord from the fifth to the twelfth weeks. This may persist until term and give rise to a congenital umbilical hernia or exomphalos.

The sex of the foetus can be seen on inspection from the fourth month onwards. In male foetuses, the testicles descend from the abdomen through the inguinal canals into the scrotum between the seventh and ninth months of pregnancy.

At birth the infant contains about 400 mg. of iron, which are present partly in the haemoglobin of the red cells of the blood and partly in the liver and tissues. Red-blood cells require iron when they are manufactured in the baby's bone marrow, liver and spleen, and as milk contains very little iron the baby is able to draw on the reserves in the liver and so avoids developing anaemia during the first few months of life.

The calcium content of the baby at birth is about 30 grammes. This is utilized chiefly in the development of the bones and tooth follicles, although calcium ions are present in the blood and in all tissue fluids. Calcium occurs in combination with phosphorus in the bones and teeth, and the new-born baby contains about 18 grammes of this substance.

Iodine is present in the thyroid gland from the sixth month of pregnancy onwards.

BEHAVIOUR OF THE FOETUS IN UTERO

Owing to the restricting space of the amniotic cavity, the foetus adopts a flexed attitude in utero, and takes up as little room as possible by bending his head and arms in front of the chest and his legs in front of the abdomen. This attitude however is not an intrinsic property of the foetus, for if there is more space available, as in cases of hydramnios, he shows no hesitation in extending his spine and limbs.

The baby functions as an independent entity after birth, and, in preparation for this, his physiological processes show marked activity during foetal life. The most important of these are as follows:

1. *Movements.* The skeletal muscles develop about the eighth week of pregnancy and foetal movements probably begin about this time, although they are not appreciated by the mother until about the seventeenth week. Up until the thirty-sixth week the movements become progressively more and more vigorous, but after this time they are less obvious.

2. *Blood circulation.* The heart begins to beat about the third week of life and the foetal circulation is then set in motion. In this way adequate oxygenation and nutrition are assured when the embryo becomes too large to be nourished by the processes of direct osmosis and diffusion. The foetal heart sounds are usually not loud enough to be heard until about the twentieth week of pregnancy.

3. *Respiration.* Respiratory movements of the lungs can be made to occur by artificial stimulation of the foetus from about the twelfth week onwards. It is doubtful if these occur so early in the normal foetus, but slight breathing movements do occur normally during the last four weeks of pregnancy. These cause liquor amnii to circulate in the trachea and bronchi.

4. *Swallowing.* This occurs during pregnancy, as is shown by the presence of lanugo in the foetal stomach and intestines. Radio-opaque material injected into the liquor is swallowed, and may be seen in the foetal stomach on subsequent X-ray examination.

The absence of swallowing in utero is thought to be one of the causes of hydramnios, as is seen in association with anencephalic monsters and infants with hydrops foetalis. Hydramnios occurs with oesophageal atresia, because although the liquor is swallowed, it cannot pass into the stomach and be absorbed and so regain the mother's circulation via the placenta.

5. *Peristalsis.* Foetal gut movements are active in pregnancy as is shown by the fact that meconium, which is coloured by bile pigments, fills the bowel from the duodenum to the rectum.

6. *Micturition.* This also is thought to be performed by the foetus during pregnancy, and to account for the urea present in the liquor amnii. In foetuses with an imperforate urethra the bladder may be distended at birth, as a result of the inability to micturate in utero. On the other hand foetal micturition is not essential, and live babies may be born at term in the complete absence of both kidneys.

7. *Hiccough.* This also is thought to occur in utero.

One function which does not take place in utero, except in states of foetal distress, is defaecation. Under normal conditions the anal canal is closed by the tone of the anal sphincters, and no meconium escapes to discolour the liquor.

THE LIQUOR AMNII

The liquor amnii is a pale straw-coloured fluid, which fills the amniotic cavity and surrounds the foetus and umbilical cord. Its specific gravity is 1006 and its reaction is slightly on the alkaline side of neutrality (pH 7·21). The quantity of liquor increases steadily as pregnancy advances, but relative to the foetus it is most abundant in mid-pregnancy; at term about 2 pints (1136 ml.) of liquor are present in normal cases.

The liquor contains certain solid constituents, namely desquamated cells from the foetus and amnion, lanugo and vernix caseosa. It is composed of 1·2 per cent solid matter dissolved in 98·8 per cent water, the constituents being as follows:

	Per cent
Protein	0·23
Glucose	0·03
Sodium Chloride	0·62
Other solids	0·32
Water	98·80
Total	100·00

In cases of diabetes mellitus the liquor may contain increased quantities of glucose.

The liquor amnii is derived from four sources:

1. Secretion by the cells of the amnion.
2. Transudation from the foetal vessels in the cord and placenta.
3. Transudation from the maternal vessels in the decidua.
4. Micturition by the foetus.

It is removed by the swallowing action of the foetus when it is absorbed into the foetal circulation and carried to the placenta. The liquor thus is not stagnant, but is being continually changed during pregnancy, i.e. there is a circulation of liquor amnii in progress during this time. Studies with radio-active substances have shown that at term 350 ml. of water in the liquor are exchanged every hour, so that the total volume is renewed every 2·9 hours. This must, therefore, be considered the time of the amniotic circulation. The sodium content of the liquor is changed in a much longer time, namely, 20·5 hours—the significance of this difference is not clear, but presumably the amniotic epithelium is more permeable to water than to sodium ions.

The functions of the liquor during pregnancy are:

1. To protect the foetus against damage from trauma to the mother's abdomen.
2. To permit foetal movements to occur.
3. To prevent adhesions forming between the foetus and the amnion.
4. To maintain the foetus at a constant temperature.
5. To equalize pressure over the foetus and cord.
6. To provide some nutritive material to the foetus derived from the small amounts that are swallowed.

During labour its functions may be considered to be:

1. To equalize the compression of the foetus by the contracting uterus.
2. To prevent excessive diminution in the size of the placental site.
3. To help impede the entry of bacteria into the uterus, after the membranes have ruptured.

THE FUNCTIONS OF THE PLACENTA

Study of the foetus would be incomplete without consideration of the functions of the placenta, for during pregnancy this organ does the work of the foetal lungs, alimentary tract, kidneys and certain ductless glands. Its chief functions may be grouped under the following headings:

1. Respiratory Function

It is through the placenta that the foetus derives its oxygen supply from the oxygenated maternal arterial blood. Oxygen (O_2) is carried to the placenta in the maternal blood in the form of oxyhaemoglobin (HbO_2). When this blood occupies the intervillous spaces, the oxyhaemoglobin splits up or dissociates into haemoglobin and oxygen (Hb and O_2).

$$\text{Maternal } HbO_2 \rightarrow \text{Reduced maternal } Hb + O_2.$$

The oxygen diffuses through the walls of the villi and the reverse action takes place in the foetal blood within the villi, the oxygen combining with the reduced foetal haemoglobin to form foetal oxyhaemoglobin.

$$\text{Reduced foetal } Hb + O_2 \rightarrow \text{Foetal } HbO_2.$$

The maternal Hb returns in the mother's veins to her lungs for re-oxygenation, whilst the foetal HbO_2 is carried in the foetal circulation to the foetal tissues. Here it dissociates, gives up oxygen to the growing cells of the tissues, and the reduced foetal Hb then returns to the placenta for re-oxygenation.

The maternal blood, however, is not such a good source of supply of oxygen as is the atmospheric air, and to compensate for this the foetal blood contains more red cells (about 7,000,000 per c. mm.) and more Hb (about 110 per cent), than are present in the mother's blood. The foetal heart action is also more rapid (about 140 beats per minute) for the same reason.

Another factor of importance is the haemoglobin of the foetus which has a slightly different chemical composition from that of the child and adult, being known as 'foetal haemoglobin' as opposed to 'adult haemoglobin'. It has the property of combining with oxygen more readily than adult haemoglobin. Curves known as Dissociation Curves may be constructed which show the amount of oxygen that combines with haemoglobin (this is known as its percentage saturation) under varying pressures; the increased avidity of foetal haemoglobin for oxygen is shown by its dissociation curve having a 'shift to the left' as compared to the dissociation curve of adult haemoglobin. This indicates that its percentage saturation is greater at the same oxygen tension. Foetal haemoglobin gradually becomes replaced by haemoglobin of the adult variety as pregnancy progresses, and at the time of delivery only about 80 per cent of the haemoglobin is foetal in type. At term the blood in the umbilical vein is about 50 per cent saturated with oxygen, whilst that in the umbilical arteries is only 15 per cent saturated.

The other respiratory function, namely the passage of carbon dioxide (CO_2) from the foetal blood to the maternal circulation also takes place through the walls of the villi. This occurs by simple diffusion, as CO_2 is much more soluble in blood than is oxygen.

2. Alimentary Function

All food products pass from the maternal to the foetal blood through the walls of the villi. The process, however, is not always one of simple diffusion, and the placenta has the power, particularly during early pregnancy when the quality of the food is more important to the developing embryo than the quantity, of breaking down complex food substances into simpler compounds and then selecting those which are required. Thus proteins are first broken down to amino-acids which are then absorbed. The selectivity of the placenta is shown by the fact that the amount of amino-acids in the foetal blood always exceeds that in the maternal circulation. Some proteins, on the other hand, pass through the placenta unchanged. Examples are antibodies and agglutinins, as may be seen in cases of erythroblastosis foetalis. Toxins and antitoxins, such as those of tetanus and diphtheria, and endocrine secretions, are also readily transmitted to the foetus.

Glucose passes freely across the placenta, although the amount present in the maternal blood is always greater than that in the foetus.

The decidua and placenta contain large quantities of glycogen. This is broken down by the placenta into glucose which is then passed on to the foetus. This is sometimes known as the glycogenic function of the placenta.

Fats and related substances (lipoids and cholesterol) pass the placental barrier slowly and with extreme difficulty. Some authorities consider they cannot pass, especially in the early months, as the placenta is impermeable to them; in this event the fat in the foetus is probably synthesized from carbohydrates in the foetal tissues.

The fat-soluble vitamins A, D and E are stored in the trophoblast cells and also pass through the placenta slowly; the water-soluble vitamins B and C however are transmitted readily. Sodium ions pass more easily as pregnancy advances, whilst calcium, phosphorus, and non-protein nitrogen are found in the foetal circulation in greater amounts than in the maternal blood. Urea, uric acid and creatinine, however, are equal in amount in both circulations and presumably pass by simple diffusion.

3. Storage Function

It has already been mentioned that the placenta stores certain food substances prior to passing them on to the foetus. Chief among these are glycogen, vitamins A and D, and iron.

4. Excretory Function

Waste metabolic substances, in addition to CO_2, pass by diffusion in the reverse direction from the foetal to the maternal blood, and are then excreted by the mother.

5. Hormone Function

The following hormones are elaborated in the placenta:

(a) *Oestrogens.* Oestrogens in the form of oestradiol are produced by the corpus luteum during the first three months of pregnancy and by the syncytium of the placenta during the final six months. They are also derived from the cortex of the suprarenal glands of both the mother and the foetus during this time, and their excretion products oestriol and oestrone are present in the urine. The amount of the former is sometimes measured and used as an index of foetal well-being.

(b) *Progesterone.* This also comes during the first three months from the corpus luteum and later from the syncytium of the placenta. Probably some is also derived from the cortex of the mother's suprarenal glands. It is produced in increasing quantities until immediately preceding the onset of labour. Its excretion product pregnanediol is present in the urine and is sometimes measured and used as an index of placental efficiency.

(c) *Chorionic Gonadotrophin.* This hormone is produced by the Langhans' cells of the cytotrophoblast from the time the blastocyst begins to embed until term. It is present in maximum quantities at the end of the second month after which it sinks to a low level in the fourth month and remains low until term. It is excreted in the urine and serves as the basis of the various animal and agglutination pregnancy tests. Its function is to stimulate the growth and activity of the corpus luteum in early pregnancy.

(d) *Relaxin.* This is a non-steroid protein hormone about which little is known. It is present during the pregnancy of certain lower mammals and has a specific action in relaxing the ligaments of joints, including the pelvic joints. The effect of this is to enlarge the capacity of the pelvis and so permit easier labour. Whether it occurs in women is not certain, but if it does it is probably elaborated by the ovary or placenta.

(e) *Adrenocorticotrophic hormone* (*ACTH*). This hormone, and possibly adrenocorticosteroid hormones, may be produced by the placenta.

6. Barrier Action

The placenta sometimes acts as a barrier and prevents harmful substances passing from the mother to the foetus. Thus the tubercle bacillus, the trypanosome, the malaria parasite and the anterior poliomyelitis virus only very rarely pass from an infected mother to give the disease to the foetus.

Unfortunately this barrier action is not very complete and the placenta is easily traversed by drugs such as morphia, pethidine and inhalation anaesthetics, by the spirochaete of syphilis, the typhoid bacillus, and by the viruses of german measles, smallpox and chicken-pox. The virus of german measles thrives well in the developing foetal tissues, and if the infected mother is two or three months pregnant, it easily penetrates the trophoblast and may give rise to congenital deformities such as cataract, deaf-mutism and congenital heart disease. The passage of rhesus antibodies to cause erythroblastosis foetalis has already been mentioned. Some substances which are beneficial to the foetus also pass through the placenta—these include penicillin, drugs employed in the treatment of syphilis, and nalorphine hydrobromide which is used to combat the respiratory depressant action of morphine and pethidine.

THE FOETAL CIRCULATION

Because the foetus derives its supply of oxygen and food from the placenta, the whole of the foetal blood has to pass through this organ, whilst the lungs and alimentary tract, being functionless during pregnancy, require only a small blood supply. The foetus in utero there-

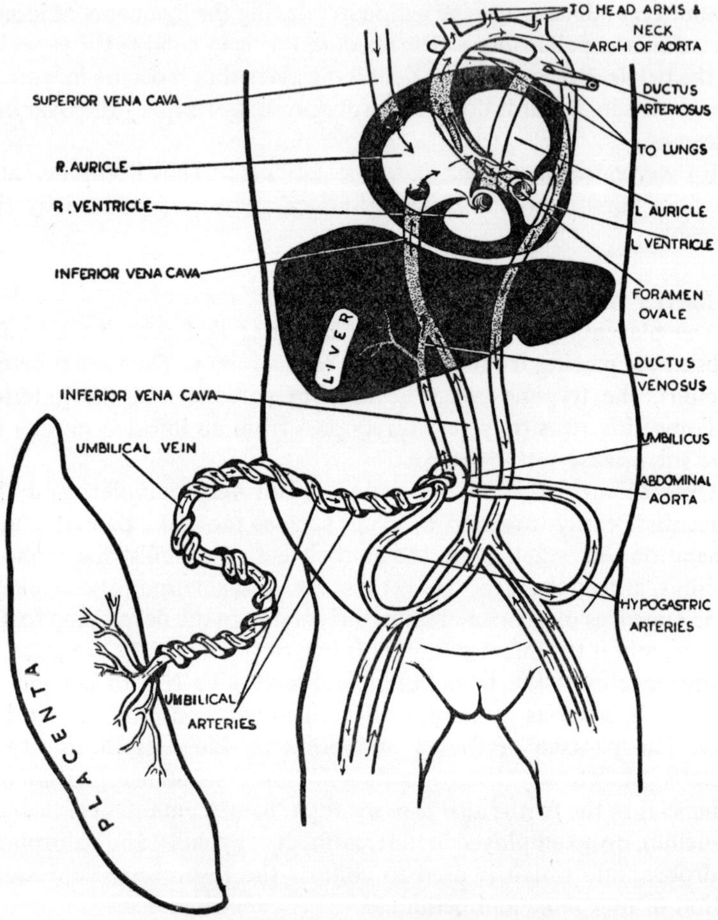

FIGURE 64. Diagram of the foetal circulation (see the following four diagrams for details)

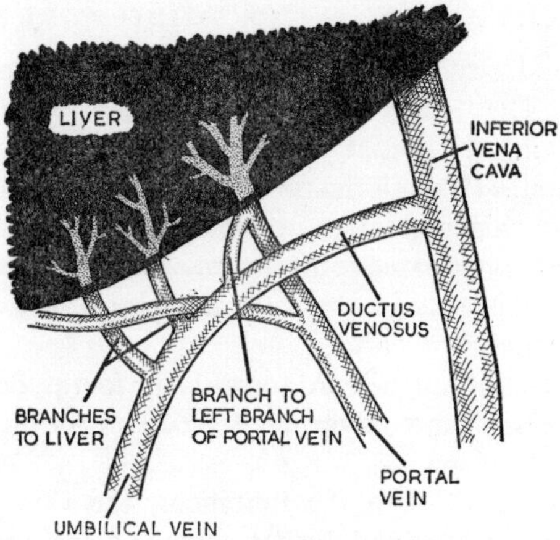

FIGURE 65. Diagram of the ductus venosus and its connections

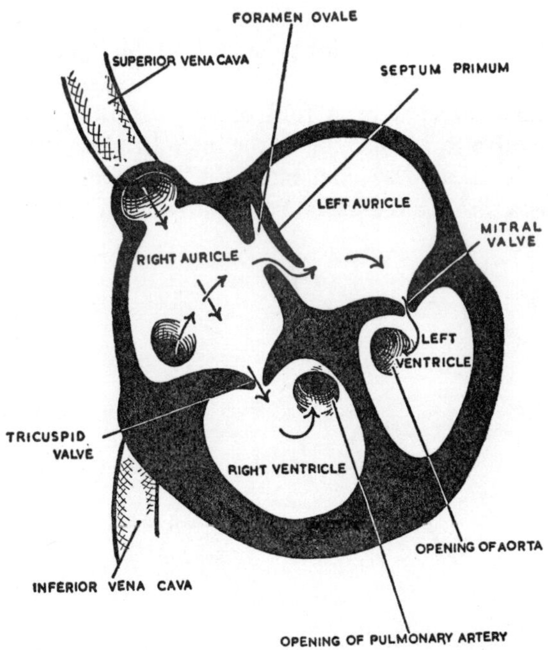

FIGURE 66. Diagram of the heart to show the formation of the foramen ovale. After birth it is sealed by the septum primum

fore has a blood circulation which differs greatly from that of its post-natal life. The details of the foetal circulation are best understood by following the course pursued by the blood as it leaves the placenta, circulates through the foetus and returns to the placenta.

The details of this circulation are as follows:

1. After being oxygenated (50 per cent saturated with oxygen) and receiving food products in the villi, the blood flows through the placenta to the umbilical cord.

2. It then passes along the cord towards the foetus, flowing through the umbilical vein. Thus oxygenated blood flows in the umbilical vein.

3. After passing through the umbilicus, the vein passes to the under surface of the liver and divides, giving off some small branches which enter the liver directly, and another branch which unites with the left branch of the portal vein and delivers blood to the liver along with the venous portal blood. The main branch, however, known as the ductus venosus, lies in a groove in the liver and joins the inferior vena cava.

4. It passes along the inferior vena cava to the right atrium of the heart.

5. It is then directed by a fold of endocardium known as the Eustachian valve to an opening in the inter-atrial septum called the foramen ovale through which it enters the left atrium.

6. It passes through the mitral valve into the left ventricle.

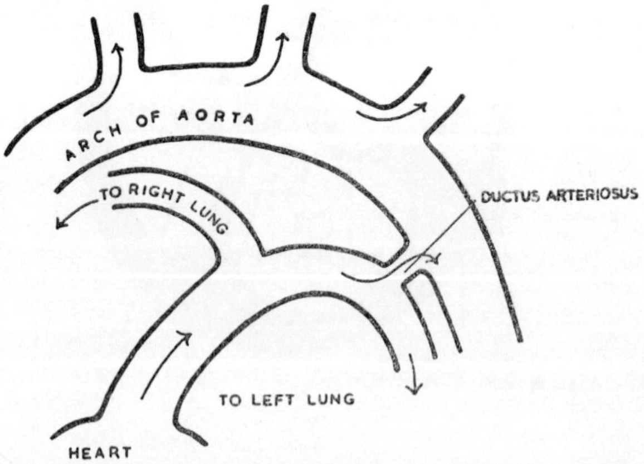

FIGURE 67. Diagram showing the position of the ductus arteriosus

7. The blood then enters the aorta, and passes along its branches to supply the head, neck and arms. This ensures that the brain, the most vital organ of the body, receives freshly oxygenated foetal blood.

8. After passing through the tissues of the head, neck and arms, the now de-oxygenated blood returns to the heart via the superior vena cava.

9. It enters the right atrium and flows through the tricuspid valve into the right ventricle. Whilst in the right atrium, this stream of impure blood crosses the stream of purified blood entering from the inferior vena cava. The special positions of the entering veins and the Eustachian valve ensure that the streams remain separate, but about 25 per cent of each flow of blood becomes mixed with the other stream.

10. From the right ventricle the de-oxygenated blood enters the trunk of the pulmonary artery.

11. Only a small stream passes through the pulmonary arteries to the functionless lungs; the major part of the blood flows through a broad channel—the ductus arteriosus—into the aorta, beyond the points of origin of the branches to the head, neck and arms.

12. The impure blood passes down the aorta and supplies the main body organs.

13. When the aorta divides into the common iliac arteries, only small streams pass down into the legs. The main streams of blood pass into the hypogastric arteries.

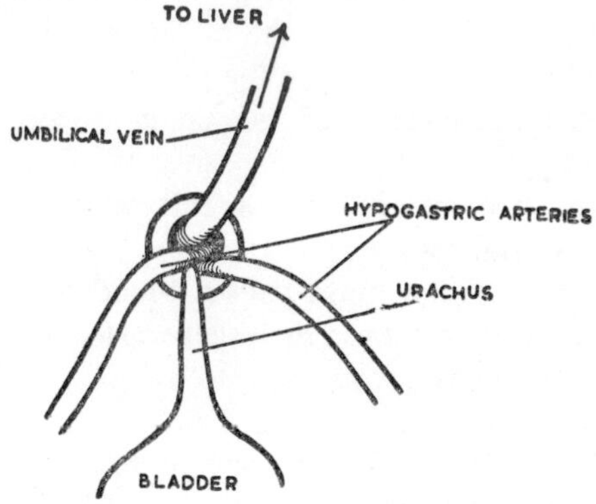

FIGURE 68. Posterior view of the foetal umbilicus, showing the entry of the umbilical vein, the exit of the hypogastric arteries, and the communication of the urachus with the apex of the bladder

14. The hypogastric arteries arise in the pelvis from the common iliac arteries and pass up the abdominal wall, converging on each side towards the umbilicus, as described in Chapter 2.

15. They pass through the umbilicus and enter the cord as the two umbilical arteries. The arteries in the cord thus transport de-oxygenated blood (about 15 per cent saturated with oxygen) back to the placenta.

16. Branches of the umbilical arteries enter the villi where re-oxygenation of the impure blood takes place.

The time taken for the whole circulation to occur is about 30 seconds.

CHANGES AT BIRTH

After birth the following changes occur:

1. When the midwife clamps the cord, the circulation through the umbilical vein ceases and the vein collapses. Its abdominal portion later becomes fibrosed to form a ligament, known as the ligamentum teres, which runs from the umbilicus to the liver. It is enclosed in a fold of peritoneum known as the falciform ligament.

2. This change leads to collapse of the ductus venosus, which in its turn becomes fibrosed later to form a ligament lying in a groove or fissure in the liver and known as the ligamentum venosum.

3. With the collapse of the umbilical vein the pressure of blood in the right atrium diminishes; with the beginning of respiration and the enhanced pulmonary circulation the pressure of blood in the left atrium increases. These changes of pressure cause a part of the heart known as the septum primum to move over the foramen ovale and seal it off; it later becomes fibrosed in this position and forms the intact adult inter-atrial septum.

4. The expansion of the lungs causes blood to flow into them through the pulmonary arteries; the ductus arteriosus consequently closes and later becomes converted into a ligament known as the ligamentum arteriosum.

5. When the blood-flow through the umbilical cord ceases the umbilical and hypogastric arteries contract and become closed. The latter vessels later become converted into ligaments in the pelvis and abdominal wall, known as the obliterated hypogastric arteries. The first few inches of these vessels, however, remain patent and become the internal iliac and superior vesical arteries.

In this way the adult circulation is produced, but the unwanted remains of the foetal circulation, which in utero functioned as large vascular channels, remain permanently present in the form of ligamentary structures.

CHAPTER 7

The Anatomy of the Foetus and its Appendages at Term

THE ANATOMY OF THE FOETUS AT TERM

The normal foetus at term weighs about seven pounds (3,200 grammes) and measures twenty inches (50 cm.) in length. It has a pale pink colour, and a rounded contour due to the liberal deposition of fat in its subcutaneous tissues. Some lanugo may still be present on the shoulders, and the hairs of the scalp are usually dark in colour and about one inch (2·5 cm.) in length. The skin is covered with the greasy excretion of the sebaceous glands known as vernix caseosa, and the nails reach to the ends of the fingers and toes.

Although at term the foetus is ready to exist independently of its mother, its shape is not the same as that of a human adult, for the head is large compared to the rest of the body, and the arms are longer than the legs, as described in Chapter 6. The process of ossification is well advanced in the bones, that of girls being slightly ahead of that of boys. Ossification centres are usually present in the lower ends of the femora, the upper ends of the tibiae and in the cuboid bones of the feet—when seen on X-ray examination these are considered to be diagnostic of a full-time foetus. The joints have a mobility greater than in later life.

The bowel is filled with meconium, a greenish-black substance with the consistency of butter. This is composed of excretions from the alimentary glands coloured with bile pigments, and contains desquamated cells from the bowel wall, and lanugo hairs from the swallowed liquor amnii.

The liver, spleen and suprarenal glands are enlarged relative to their size in the adult. In males the testicles have reached the scrotum. In females the labia majora are full and rounded due to the deposition of subcutaneous fat, the vaginal walls are well cornified and the uterus is actually larger than that of the young girl. These latter changes are due to the influence of sex hormones which have passed into the foetus from the placenta; after birth these organs retrogress and do not develop further until the young girl manufactures her own sex hormones at the time of puberty.

THE FOETAL SKULL AT TERM

The most important part of the foetus at term, from the midwife's point of view, is the skull. As this is both the largest and hardest part of the foetus, it gives rise to many of the difficulties which may occur during the process of birth; a knowledge therefore of the cranial anatomy is essential.

Bones

The vault of the skull is composed of five bones, with two others entering into the formation of its lateral walls. All these bones are ossified in pre-existing membrane. They may be described as follows:

(i) *The two frontal bones* extend from the upper borders of the orbits to the coronal suture. They are large bones, roughly square in shape, and are curved as they cover the frontal lobes of the brain.

(ii) *The two parietal bones* lie behind the frontal bones, extending from the coronal suture in front to the lambdoid suture behind. They are the largest of the cranial bones, also roughly square in shape, and curved as they lie over the parietal lobes of the brain. In the centre of each is situated a bony eminence which is known as the parietal eminence.

(iii) *The occipital bone* is a single bone lying below the parietal bones, from which it is separated by the lambdoid suture. It is roughly triangular in shape, and covers the occipital lobes of the brain and the cerebellum. In its central part is situated a small eminence, the external occipital protuberance (or inion), commonly referred to simply as the occiput. On its internal surface is similarly placed another bony point, the internal occipital protuberance, to which folds of dura mater are attached, as described below.

In its lower part this bone forms the margins of the foramen magnum, through which the lower part of the brain and spinal cord become continuous; it also articulates with the atlas, or first cervical vertebra.

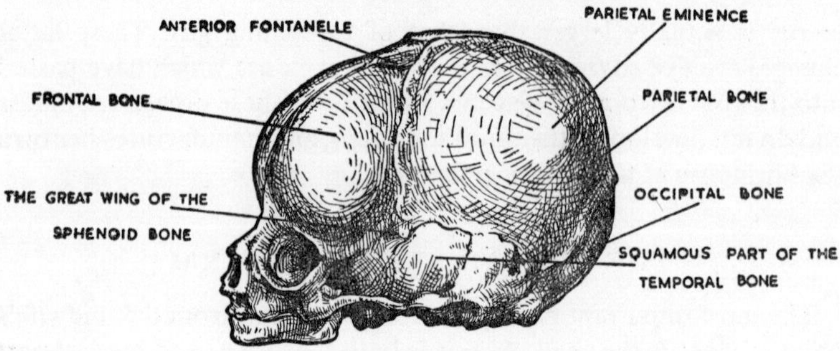

FIGURE 69. Lateral view of the foetal skull

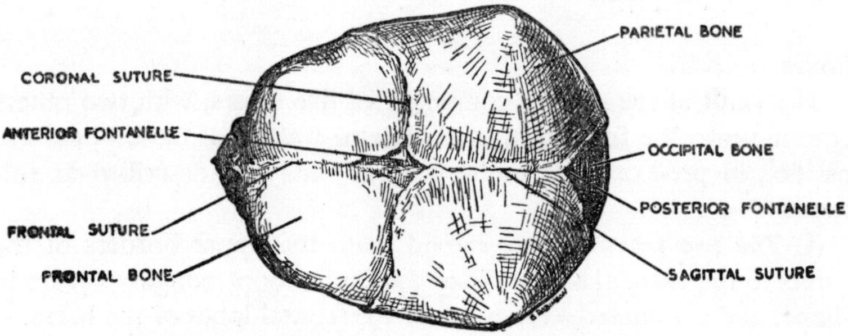

FIGURE 70. Superior view of the foetal skull

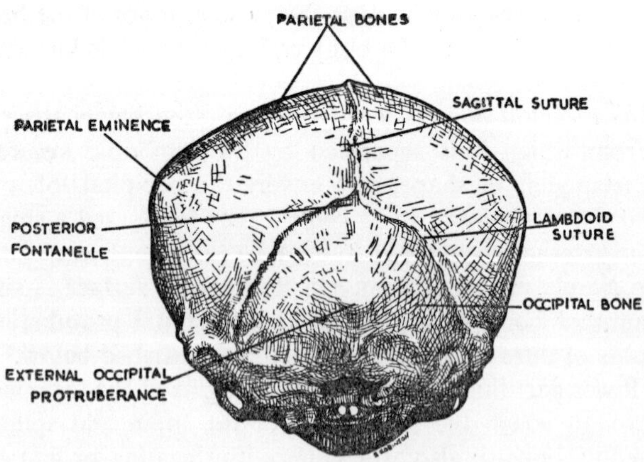

FIGURE 71. Posterior view of the foetal skull

(iv) *The two temporal bones* form part of the side walls of the foetal skull. The squamous portion of the temporal bone lies below the parietal bone in front of the ear, whilst the mastoid portion of the same bone lies behind the ear.

(v) *The great wings of the sphenoid bone* occupy a small area between the frontal bones in front and the squamous part of the temporal bones behind.

Sutures

The parts of the skull where the bones lie alongside each other are known as the sutures of the skull. The sutures are composed of a fibrous membrane, and they allow some of the bones to overlap each other during the process of moulding at the time of birth. As ossification proceeds after birth, the bones gradually fuse together, with the result that the membranous sutures disappear and a solid bony cranium enclosing and protecting the brain is formed.

The chief sutures are as follows:

(i) *The frontal suture or metopic suture* runs between the frontal bones, extending from the root of the nose (or nasion) below, to the anterior fontanelle above.

(ii) *The sagittal suture* lies between the two parietal bones and runs from the anterior fontanelle in front to the posterior fontanelle behind.

(iii) *The coronal suture* runs transversely across the head, lying between the frontal bones in front and the parietal bones behind. It enters the anterior fontanelle at its lateral angles.

(iv) *The lambdoid suture* passes obliquely across the posterior part of the skull, lying between the two parietal bones above and the occipital bone below. It passes from the mastoid part of each temporal bone upwards and inwards and joins the posterior fontanelle.

Fontanelles

These are the areas of membrane lying between the cranial bones at the points of junction of the sutures. Two are of great obstetrical importance:

(i) *The anterior fontanelle or bregma.* This is a lozenge-shaped area, lying between the two parietal and two frontal bones, measuring $1\frac{1}{2}$ inches (3·8 cm.) in length and $\frac{3}{4}$ inch (19 mm.) in breadth. It has four angles, into each of which runs a suture; thus the frontal suture enters the fontanelle anteriorly, the sagittal suture posteriorly, and the coronal suture at the lateral angles.

It becomes smaller after birth and disappears when it is completely ossified at the age of eighteen months.

(ii) *The posterior fontanelle or lambda.* This is a small triangular-shaped space lying between the two parietal bones and the occipital bone. It has three angles; into the anterior angle runs the sagittal suture, whilst the two parts of the lambdoid suture run into the lateral angles.

It becomes ossified when the baby is aged two months.

In addition to these large fontanelles, four small ones are present in the lateral walls of the foetal skull:

(i) Two temporal fontanelles, situated at the extremities of the coronal suture.

(ii) Two mastoid fontanelles, placed at the terminal points of the lambdoid suture.

These have no obstetrical significance.

Regions of the Skull

The following are the regions of the skull which are of most importance:

(i) *The vertex* is the area of the skull which lies between the anterior fontanelle in front, the posterior fontanelle behind, and the two parietal eminences laterally.

(ii) *The sinciput or brow* lies between the supra-orbital ridges below and the coronal suture and bregma above.

(iii) *The occiput* is the part of the skull lying below the lambdoid suture and posterior fontanelle. Sometimes this area is referred to as the occipital pole, and the term occiput is then restricted to the external occipital protuberance.

(iv) *The face* is the part of the skull which lies below the level of the supra-orbital ridges.

Diameters

The presenting diameters of the foetal skull are important because they are the distances which the birth canal must stretch to allow passage of the head during delivery. In all cases the maximum transverse diameter is the bi-parietal diameter, but the maximum antero-posterior diameter varies according to the degree of flexion or extension of the head. The maximum antero-posterior diameter thus differs according to the presentation of the foetus, as is shown in the following table:

Presentation	A-P Diameter	Length in inches	Length in cm.
Vertex	Sub-occipito-bregmatic	3¾	9·5
Breech (after-coming-head)	Sub-occipito-frontal	4	10·1
Bregmatic (or occipito-posterior position)	Occipito-frontal	4½	11·4
Face	Sub-mento-bregmatic	3¾	9·5
Brow	Mento-vertical	5¼	13·3

(i) *The sub-occipito-bregmatic diameter* runs from the junction of the scalp with the back of the neck (below the position of the occiput) to the bregma.

(ii) *The sub-occipito-frontal diameter* passes from the junction of the scalp with the back of the neck to the mid-point of the frontalsuture.

(iii) *The occipito-frontal diameter* passes from the external occipital protuberance or inion to the root of the nose or nasion.

(iv) *The sub-mento-bregmatic diameter* runs from the junction of the chin and the neck to the bregma.

(v) *The mento-vertical diameter* extends from the point of the chin to the centre of the vertex. It is the longest diameter of the foetal skull.

(vi) *The sub-mento-vertical diameter* runs from the junction of the chin and the neck to the centre of the vertex and measures 4½ inches (11·4 cm.).

(vii) *The bi-parietal diameter* extends between the parietal eminences and measures 3¾ inches (9·5 cm.).

(viii) *The bi-temporal diameter* runs between the two extremities of the coronal suture, and is 3¼ inches (8·3 cm.) in length.

(ix) *The bi-mastoid diameter* lies between the tips of the mastoid processes and measures 3 inches (7·6 cm.).

Three further diameters of the foetus are important:

(i) *The bis-acromial diameter* extends between the acromial processes of the scapulae. It is 4¾ inches (12·0 cm.) in length.

(ii) *The bi-trochanteric diameter* runs between the greater trochanters of the femora, and measures 4 inches (10·1 cm.) in length.

(iii) *The bis-iliac diameter* runs between the points farthermost apart on the iliac crests. It also measures 4 inches (10·1 cm.).

Circumferences

Certain circumferences of the foetus are also of importance:

(i) *The sub-occipito-bregmatic circumference* is measured around the ends of the sub-occipito-bregmatic diameter, and is the girdle of contact of the foetal skull in vertex presentations. It measures 11¾ inches (29·2 cm.) in length.

(ii) *The occipito-frontal circumference* is measured around the ends of the occipito-frontal diameter, and is the girdle of contact in face-to-pubes deliveries. It is 14 inches (35·6 cm.) in length.

(iii) *The mento-vertical circumference* is similarly measured around the ends of the mento-vertical diameter, and is the girdle of contact in brow presentations. It is the largest circumference of the foetal skull, measuring 15 inches (38·0 cm.) in length.

(iv) *The chest circumference.* The greatest circumference around the chest measures 13¼ inches (33·6 cm.) in length.

(v) *The neck circumference*. This measures 7½ inches (19 cm.).

Moulding

During the process of moulding the size of the foetal skull is reduced by overlapping of the vault bones. Thus the edges of the frontal and occipital bones pass under the edges of the parietal bones, and the posterior parietal passes similarly under the anterior parietal. The frontal bones do not override because they are fixed at the root of the nose. In addition to these changes, the shape of the skull alters and the engaging diameters distending the birth canal become shortened. To compensate for this the diameter at right angles to the engaging diameter, lying in the axis of the pelvis, becomes correspondingly lengthened. The actual diameters which change in this way vary according to the attitude of the head, which differs with each presentation, as shown in the following table:

Presentation	*Shortened Diameter*	*Lengthened Diameter*
Normal vertex	Sub-occipito-bregmatic	Mento-vertical
Breech (after-coming head)	Sub-occipito-frontal	Sub-mento-vertical
Bregmatic (or occipito-posterior)	Occipito-frontal	Sub-mento-bregmatic
Face	Sub-mento-bregmatic	Occipito-frontal
Brow	Mento-vertical	Sub-occipito-bregmatic

THE SCALP

The scalp of the foetus consists of five layers, placed in the following order:

(i) The skin.

(ii) A layer of subcutaneous tissue containing blood-vessels and hair follicles. It is this part of the scalp which may become oedematous and form the caput succedaneum associated with difficult or prolonged labour.

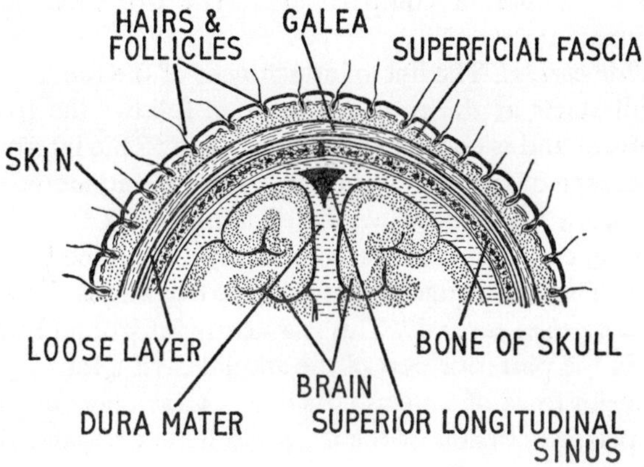

FIGURE 72. Diagram showing the layers of the scalp

(iii) A layer of tendon, covering the vertex, which connects the frontalis muscle in the sinciput with the occipitalis muscle in the occiput. This is known as the galea.

(iv) A loose layer of areolar tissue, which permits limited movement of the scalp to occur over the skull.

(v) The pericranium. This is the periosteum of the cranial bones which covers their outer surfaces, and is adherent to their edges. Bleeding which may occur between the bone and the pericranium during labour forms a swelling known as a cephalhaematoma. This is limited in shape to that of the bone over which it lies, owing to this attachment of the pericranium to the bony edges.

THE INTERNAL ANATOMY OF THE SKULL

In addition to the pericranium which covers the external surface of the vault bones, there is a similar membrane which lines their internal surface. Inside the skull, however, this is composed of two layers, an outer periosteal layer which is adherent to the bones themselves, and an inner meningeal layer which covers the outer surface of the brain, and is known as the dura mater. This latter membrane not only covers the whole brain but also sends fibrous partitions dipping in between the different portions of the brain, to divide up the interior of the skull into a number of compartments. The two most prominent partitions are:

(i) *The falx cerebri.* The line of attachment of the falx to the inside of the skull starts at the root of the nose, follows the frontal and sagittal sutures and is continued in the midline to the internal occipital protuberance of the occipital bone. From this attachment a vertical fold of dura hangs downwards, dividing the cavity of the skull into two equal compartments each of which is occupied by a cerebral hemisphere. The lower edge of this fold lies free and is sickle-shaped.

(ii) *The tentorium cerebelli.* This is a nearly horizontal fold of dura which lies in the posterior part of the cranial cavity, forming the roof of the posterior fossa of the skull. Its line of attachment can be traced along the petrous portion of the temporal bone on each side, and is continued across the occipital bone by a horizontal line which connects the posterior ends of the temporal bones and passes through the internal occipital protuberance. From this attachment the tentorium passes forwards and inwards and is attached to the clinoid processes of the sphenoid bone. It separates the two cerebral hemispheres above from the cerebellum below, over which it forms a domed tent-like covering.

The posterior part of the falx is attached to the upper surface of the tentorium along its middle line. Immediately in front of the point of junction of the falx and tentorium an arch is formed, through which the brain stem passes from the cerebral hemispheres to become continuous with the medulla oblongata and the spinal cord.

These portions of the dura mater are of importance in obstetrics, because large veins or sinuses, which drain blood from the brain, pass inside them on their way to become the jugular veins of the neck. Those of chief importance are:

(i) The superior longitudinal sinus, which passes along the line of attachment of the falx, running from the root of the nose to the internal occipital protuberance.

(ii) The inferior longitudinal sinus, which runs in the lower border of the falx from before backwards, ending at the point of junction with the tentorium cerebelli.

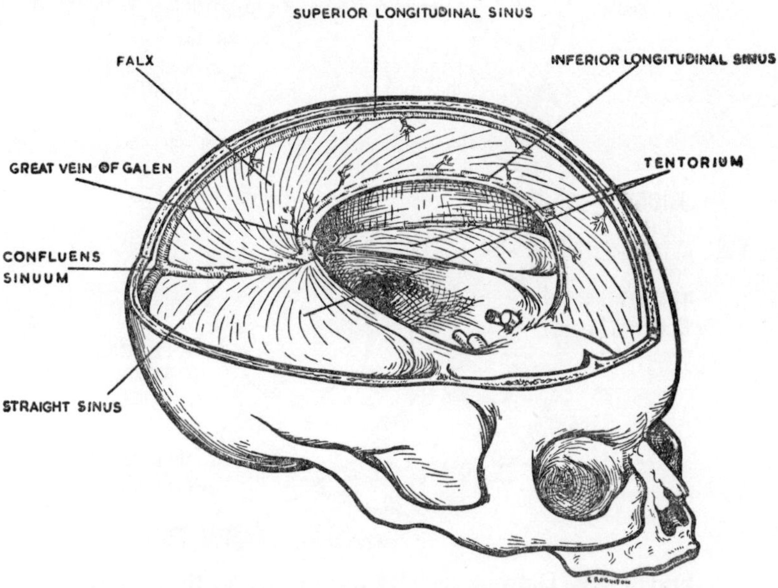

FIGURE 73. View of interior of skull, showing the falx cerebri, the tentorium cerebelli and venous sinuses

(iii) The straight sinus, which is the continuation of the inferior longitudinal sinus which passes backwards, along the line of junction of the falx and tentorium, to unite with the posterior end of the superior longitudinal sinus. This point of junction of the sinuses opposite the internal occipital protuberance is known as the confluens sinuum.

(iv) The great vein of Galen, or great internal cerebral vein, which is made up of tributaries issuing from the brain substance. It passes backwards from the surface of the brain to join the straight sinus, at the point where this becomes continuous with the inferior longitudinal sinus.

(v) From the confluens sinuum the united sinuses pass on each side of the skull along the line of attachment of the tentorium cerebelli to the occipital bone, where they are known as the lateral sinuses. They then emerge from the skull to become the internal jugular veins of the neck.

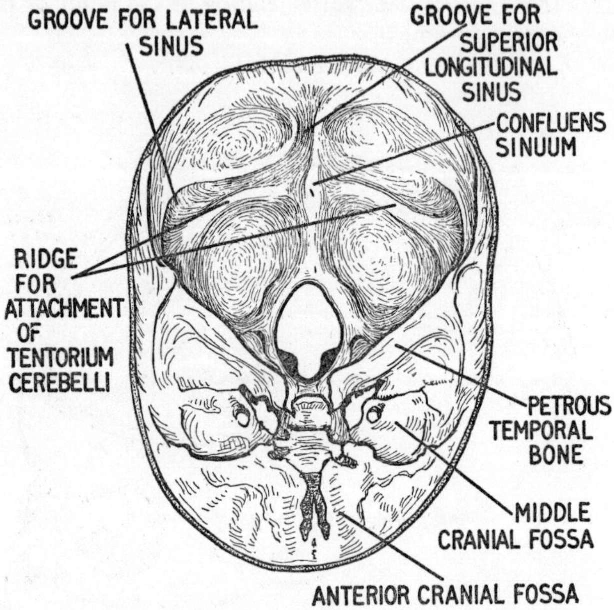

FIGURE 73a. Drawing showing the grooves for the sinuses on the inner aspect of the occipital bone

When moulding occurs at the time of delivery, the falx and tentorium and their contained sinuses are stretched. If such moulding is excessive in degree or rapid in occurrence, the membranes and the sinuses are likely to rupture; intracranial haemorrhage then occurs which may seriously affect the health of the foetus, or may even kill it outright. Such tears occur mostly in the tentorium near its attachment to the falx and are called tentorial tears. The sinuses most frequently involved in this injury are:

(i) The great vein of Galen, which becomes torn off at its point of junction with the straight sinus.

(ii) The straight sinus, which may be involved in deep tentorial tears.

(iii) The inferior longitudinal sinus, which may be torn in tears affecting the falx.

THE UMBILICAL CORD AT TERM

The umbilical cord at term is about 22 inches (56 cm.) in length, and extends normally from the centre of the placenta to the umbilicus. It is of a dull white colour, and varies in thickness from $\frac{1}{2}$ to $\frac{3}{4}$ inches (1·3 to 1·9 cm.). It is composed of a jelly-like material known as Wharton's jelly, and is covered by a layer of stratified cubical cells which are continuous with the foetal epidermis at one end of the cord, and the amniotic epithelium at the other.

It contains the following structures:

1. *One large umbilical vein.* Oxygenated blood flows through this vein from the placenta to the foetus. It contains no valves.

2. *Two umbilical arteries.* These are the continuation of the hypogastric arteries, which carry de-oxygenated blood from the foetus to the placenta. These wind around the vein in a clockwise manner about ten times as they pass along the cord. They have no internal elastic lamina and thick muscular walls which enable them to contract down and stop bleeding when the cord is severed after birth. This is of great importance in animals, where, of course, the cord is not ligated.

3. *The vitelline duct.* This small vestigial structure is the remains of the yolk sac. It passes through the umbilicus and in early embryonic life communicates with the gut, as described in Chapter 5.

4. *The allantois.* This is another small vestigial structure which passes through the umbilicus. In the early stages of development it is continuous with the urachus and the apex of the bladder; this state very rarely persists until term when the bladder opens to the exterior through the umbilicus.

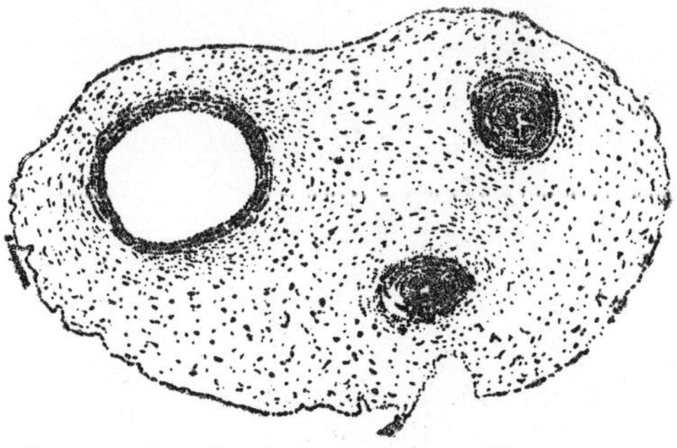

FIGURE 74. Section of the umbilical cord

The cord is not always of uniform thickness. There are sometimes present local proliferations of Wharton's jelly, which are known as false knots. On some occasions these knots may contain a loop of vessels. True knots, due to foetal movements in the liquor, are also sometimes found.

The cord is fairly strong, and will support a weight of 8 lb. (3,628 grammes) before it ruptures.

THE PLACENTA AT TERM

When the normal placenta is inspected after delivery, it is seen to be a circular flat organ, measuring about 8 inches (20·2 cm.) in diameter and 25 inches (62·5 cm.) in circumference. It is about 1 inch (2·5 cm.) in thickness at the centre, and slightly thinner at the edge. It weighs approximately 1 lb. (453 grammes), or one-sixth of the weight of the foetus. The chorion is continuous with the placenta at its edge. It is derived from the chorion frondosum of the trophoblast.

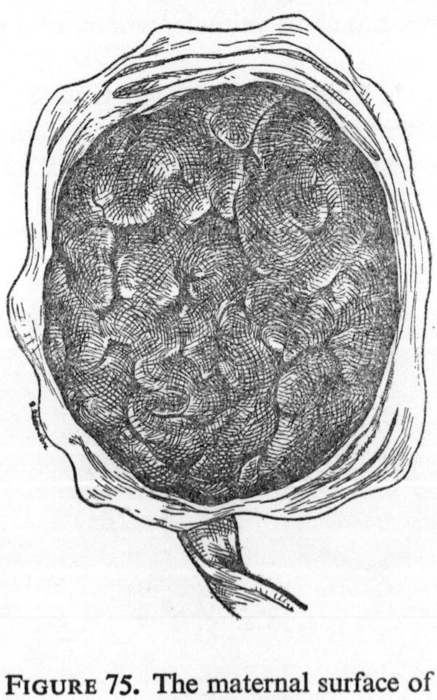

FIGURE 75. The maternal surface of the placenta

It has two surfaces:

(i) *The maternal surface.* This is the surface which is attached to the decidua basalis of the uterus during pregnancy. It is deep red in colour and is divided by deep grooves or sulci into about twenty lobes which are known as cotyledons. This part of the placenta is made up of masses of arborescent villi, and the red colour is due to the blood contained in the villi and in the intervillous spaces. The actual blood-vessels themselves cannot be seen on this surface by the naked eye.

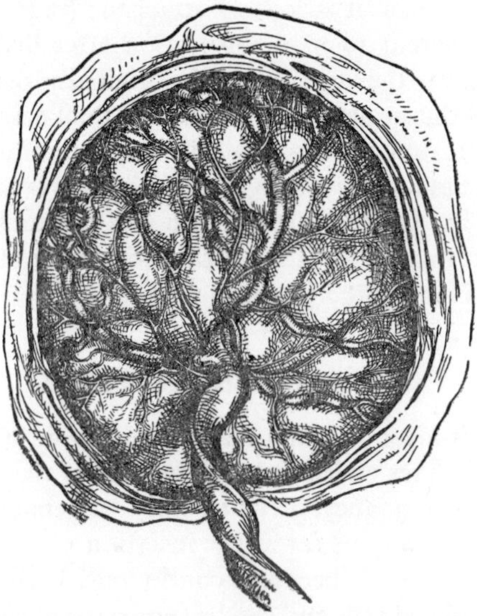

FIGURE 76. The foetal surface of the placenta

Greyish-coloured plaques may be observed attached to the surface of the cotyledons and lying between them in the sulci; these are parts of the superficial decidua, which in the sulci form decidual septa. Fibrin is often deposited on the surface of the villi, and this may in places undergo calcification; these changes impart to the fingers a gritty sensation on palpation.

(ii) *The foetal surface.* This part of the placenta lies adjacent to the amniotic cavity during pregnancy, and is therefore lined by amnion which can be stripped off it as far as the insertion of the cord. The cord is normally attached to the centre of this surface, and from its site of attachment the foetal vessels radiate out in all directions towards the edge of the placenta. The arteries and veins frequently cross each other as they pass towards the periphery, repeatedly dividing in their course, and so becoming smaller in size. They finally disappear from sight by passing deep into the substance of the placenta where they enter the villi to be distributed to all their branches.

THE CHORION AT TERM

The chorion is a rough fibrous opaque membrane which is continuous with the placenta at its edge. It lines the decidua vera of the uterine cavity to which it is loosely attached; fragments of decidua may be seen adherent to it on inspection after delivery. Its inner surface is lined by the amnion. It is originally derived from the chorion laeve of the trophoblast. At term its thickness varies between 0·2 mm. and 0·02 mm.; microscopically it is found to consist of four layers of tissue, but it contains no blood-vessels, lymphatics or nerves.

The chorion has little tensile strength and ruptures easily, so that retention of part or whole of the chorion within the uterus sometimes occurs after delivery of the placenta.

THE AMNION AT TERM

The amnion is a tough shiny membrane devoid of blood-vessels, lymphatics and nerves which lines the interior of the chorion and the placenta during pregnancy. It can gently be separated from these structures after delivery as far as the insertion of the cord, with the outer surface of which it becomes continuous. It consists of fibrous tissue lined by cubical cells and can be shown to consist of five distinct layers. Its thickness varies from 0·02 mm. to 0·5 mm. The lining cells probably secrete the liquor amnii which fills the amniotic cavity and surrounds the foetus during pregnancy. The amnion is much stronger than the chorion, and is retained within the uterus after delivery only infrequently.

CHAPTER 8

Maternal Changes During Pregnancy

During the course of pregnancy marked changes take place in the anatomical structure and physiological processes of the mother. The most outstanding of these is the growth which occurs in the uterus, but practically all the systems of the body participate in changes during this time.

CHANGES IN THE GENITAL TRACT

The Uterus

1. THE BODY OF THE UTERUS

Changes in Size

As pregnancy advances the uterus grows from its normal size of 3 inches in length, 2 inches in width and 1 inch in depth (7·6 × 5·1 × 2·5 cm.), until at term it is 12 inches long, 9 inches wide and 8 inches deep (30·4 × 22·8 × 20·2 cm.). The weight of the uterus also increases from 2 ounces to 2 pounds (56 grammes to 906 grammes). During the same time its walls become thinner and their original thickness of ½ inch is reduced to ⅓ inch by term (13 mm. to 8 mm.).

Changes in Shape

In early pregnancy when the blastocyst embeds in the decidua of the upper part of the uterine body, the muscle walls of the uterus become softened and increased in length so that the cavity of the uterus is enlarged. This makes it possible for the blastocyst to increase in size during the course of its development. Whilst the uterus is enlarging in this way, its shape becomes modified. At the beginning of pregnancy it is a pear-shaped organ; when the end of the third month is reached it becomes globular, but after the fifth month returns to a pyriform contour, which it maintains until term.

These alterations in the shape of the uterus are due to varying rates of growth which occur in its different regions. The part of the uterus first to enlarge is the upper part of the body which contains the blastocyst; it becomes uniformly enlarged and is called the upper segment of the uterus. At the same time growth occurs in the lowest part of the body of the uterus, which is known as the isthmus. As this does not normally contain the blastocyst it does not become wider, but merely increases in length, growing from about 7 mm. to 25 mm. By the time pregnancy is advanced to two months, the enlarged upper part of the uterus is continuous with the elongated isthmus, which in its turn continues into the relatively unchanged cervix below. The

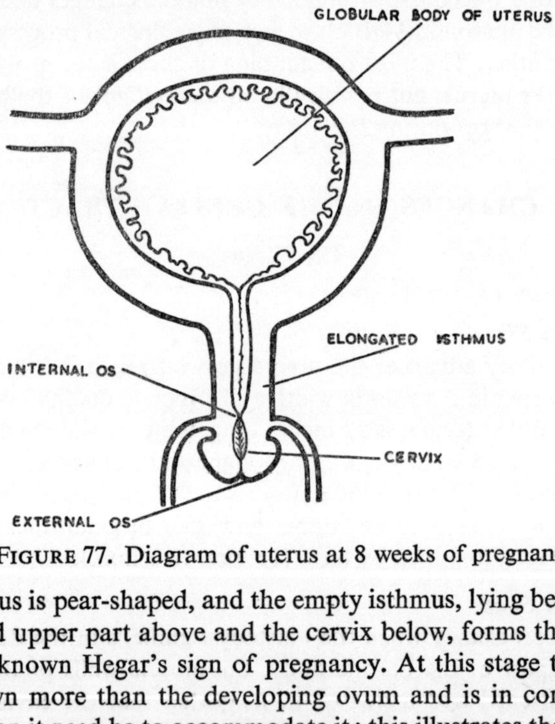

FIGURE 77. Diagram of uterus at 8 weeks of pregnancy

uterus thus is pear-shaped, and the empty isthmus, lying between the expanded upper part above and the cervix below, forms the basis of the well-known Hegar's sign of pregnancy. At this stage the uterus has grown more than the developing ovum and is in consequence larger than it need be to accommodate it; this illustrates the fact that the uterine enlargement is not directly due to the presence of the blastocyst, but is dependent upon the hormonal stimulus of oestrogens.

When the end of the third month of pregnancy is reached the amnion expands to line the chorion and the gestation sac fills the cavity of the upper segment of the uterus. The elongated isthmus then unfolds, as it were, and receives the lower pole of the developing

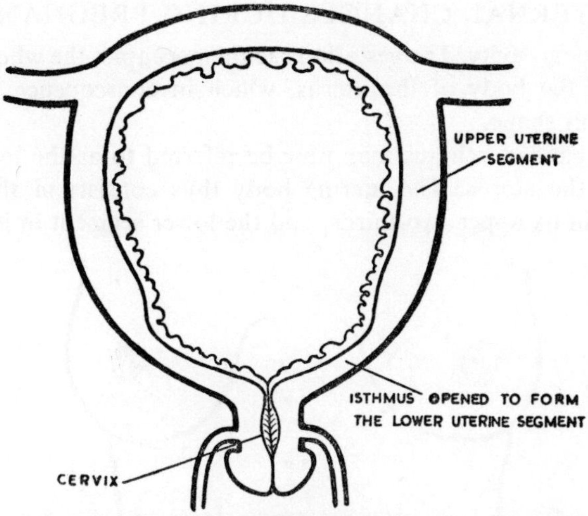

FIGURE 78. Diagram of uterus at 12 weeks of pregnancy

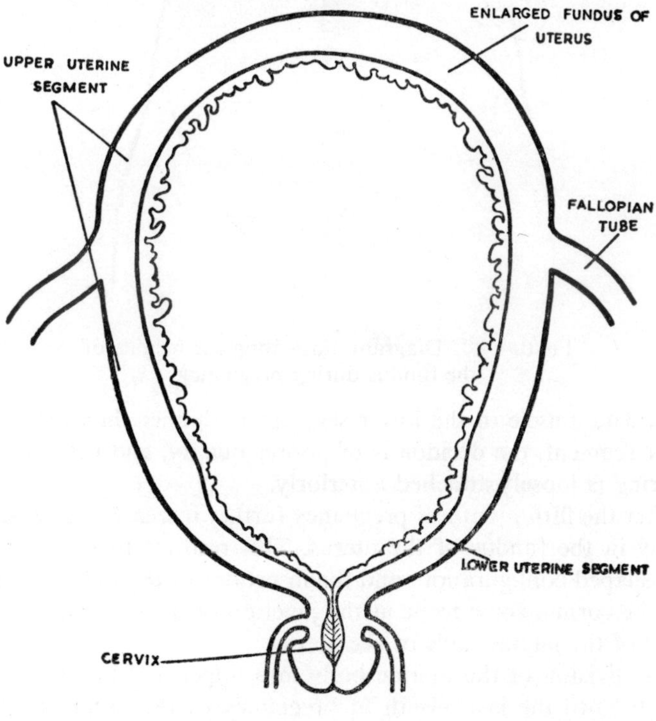

FIGURE 79. Diagram of uterus at 30 weeks of pregnancy.
(Not drawn to scale)

ovum into its cavity. The gestation sac then occupies the whole of the cavity of the body of the uterus, which in consequence becomes globular in shape.

The expanded isthmus may now be referred to as the lower segment of the uterus. The uterine body thus consists of the upper segment in its upper two-thirds, and the lower segment in its lowest

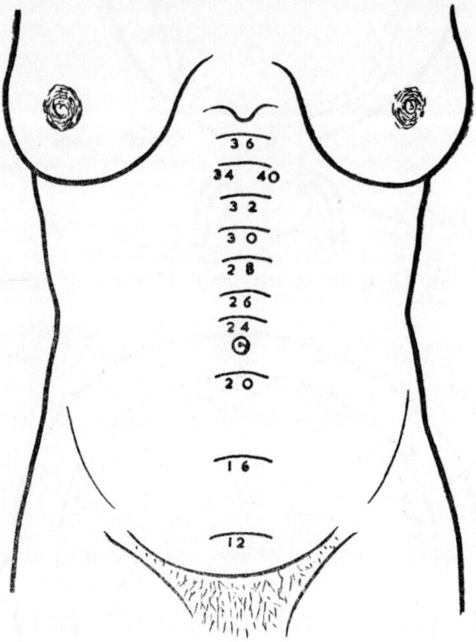

FIGURE 80. Diagram illustrating the heights of the fundus during pregnancy

third. The muscle in the lower segment is thinner than that of the upper segment, the decidua is of poorer quality, and the peritoneal covering is loosely attached anteriorly.

After the fifth month of pregnancy further increase in size occurs, chiefly in the fundus of the uterus. This restores to the uterus its pear-shaped configuration, and the insertions of the Fallopian tubes into the cornua come to lie at the junction of the upper and middle thirds of the lateral walls of the uterus.

The division of the uterine body into upper and lower segments persists until the last month of pregnancy or the onset of labour, when the cervix becomes 'taken up' and incorporated into the lower segment. The lower segment of the uterus during pregnancy thus consists solely of the isthmus; during labour it comprises both the isthmus and the cervix.

Clinical Observations of the Growing Uterus

The enlargement of the uterus may be detected clinically, as is illustrated in Fig. 80.

The fundus of the uterus is first palpable above the upper border of the pubic symphysis at the twelfth week of pregnancy. It reaches a finger's-breadth below the level of the umbilicus at 20 weeks, and gains a position midway between these points at 16 weeks.

By the 24th week, the uterus has risen to a finger's-breadth above the umbilicus, thus passing through the level of this structure at the 22nd week.

By the 36th week, the fundus reaches the level of the ensiform cartilage, gaining a point midway between this structure and the umbilicus at the 30th week. If these two distances be divided into thirds, the height of the fundus at the 26th and 28th weeks will be determined above the umbilicus, and at the 32nd and 34th weeks below the ensiform cartilage.

After the 36th week the height of the fundus depends upon diverse factors, such as the engagement of the presenting part, the tone of the muscles of the abdominal wall and the degree of uterine obliquity.

It should be remembered that these levels are only approximations to the truth as many varying factors come into play in particular patients. Thus the umbilicus and ensiform cartilage vary slightly in position in individual patients, and weak abdominal muscles may allow the uterus to become anteverted instead of rising erect in the abdomen.

Changes in the Uterine Muscle Cells

The enlargement of the body of the uterus during pregnancy is due to two factors: a process of actual growth which occurs during the first 5 months, and a process of stretch which takes place after this time. The muscle growth occurs in two ways:

(i) The actual muscle cells enlarge, increasing in length about 10 times, and in width about 3 times. This process is known as hypertrophy.

(ii) New muscle cells make their appearance and grow alongside the original muscle cells. This is called hyperplasia.

As the muscle fibres of the upper segment increase they become arranged into three layers:

(i) An outermost longitudinal layer, which is continuous with the muscle fibres in the uterine ligaments. This layer begins in the anterior wall of the upper segment, passes up over the fundus and down the posterior wall. It is by the contraction and retraction of this layer of muscle that the foetus is expelled from the uterus during labour.

(ii) A middle oblique layer, in which the muscle fibres are arranged in a criss-cross manner. These muscle cells surround the uterine blood-vessels in figure-of-eight patterns, and by their retraction after separation of the placenta during labour, they compress them and help to prevent post-partum haemorrhage. They are sometimes referred to as the living ligatures of the uterus.

(iii) An innermost circular layer. This is the weakest of the three layers and the muscle fibres pass transversely around the uterus deep to the decidua. They are most developed around the openings of the Fallopian tubes and in the lower segment.

The wall of the lower segment is thinner than that of the upper segment and consists mostly of circular fibres.

Other Changes in the Uterus

The normal anteversion and anteflexion of the uterus disappear after the twelfth week of pregnancy, and the uterus becomes erect as it rises in the abdomen. It often inclines to the right, producing what is known as the right obliquity of the uterus. It also rotates to the right as pregnancy advances. These changes are probably brought about by the pressure of the pelvic colon which is situated in the left side of the pelvis.

The arteries, veins and lymphatics supplying the uterus are all greatly enlarged during pregnancy. The tortuosities of the uterine arteries become straightened out as the growth of the uterus progresses. The main venous drainage is via the ovarian veins.

The uterine ligaments, which contain smooth muscle, become thickened during pregnancy, as a result of the increased growth of the muscle fibres.

The changes that occur in the endometrium during pregnancy are described in Chapter 5.

2. The Cervix

The cervix maintains a constant length of one inch (2·5 cm.) during pregnancy. However, it increases slightly in width, and becomes much softer after the third month. This is due to its increased vascularity, to the relaxing effect of progesterone, to the liquefaction of the collagen, and to a great proliferation of the cervical mucosa and racemose glands. These glands excrete mucus to form a mucous plug, known as the operculum, which occupies the cervical canal during pregnancy. It functions as a protective device and prevents the entry of harmful agents into the uterus during this time.

When examined through a speculum, the cervix is seen to have a lilac colour during pregnancy.

The Physiology of the Uterus during Pregnancy

The function of the uterus during pregnancy is to accommodate the foetus and its appendages. In order to effect this efficiently the uterus not only has to grow and enlarge, as already described, but it must also at the same time become relaxed so that it does not expel the embryo before the time of delivery arrives.

The necessary growth occurs as a result of stimulation by oestrogenic hormones, which are derived from the corpus luteum for the first three months of pregnancy, and from the placenta for the remaining six months. In cases of extra-uterine pregnancy, marked growth of the uterine muscle occurs as a result of this oestrogenic stimulation, although the ovum is not inside the uterus.

The relaxation is brought about by progesterone, which is derived from the same sources. It also stimulates the conversion of the endometrium into the decidua and enables embedding of the ovum to become established.

The uterus however is not completely relaxed throughout pregnancy. From the eighth week onwards periodic waves of contraction pass over it; they last for about a minute and recur at five to ten minute intervals. They are called the intermittent contractions of Braxton Hicks. They are quite painless and the patient is unaware of their presence. They probably have no function at this time, but are part of the physiological growth process of the uterine muscle, in preparation for the role the uterus will play during labour. Towards the end of pregnancy they become stronger and more frequent, and are responsible then for the taking up of the cervix when this occurs during the last month of pregnancy. When labour starts they are further increased and become true labour contractions. During pregnancy they raise the intra-uterine pressure from 7 to about 18 mm. Hg., which is below the pain threshold of 25 mm. Hg. This threshold however is exceeded when labour contractions begin and the patient then experiences discomfort or pain.

The Vagina

The vagina grows slightly during pregnancy and develops a larger lumen. It becomes very vascular and in consequence assumes a lilac hue. The vaginal fluid becomes more acid at this time.

The Vulva

The labia minora become pigmented during pregnancy and the vulva as a whole appears lilac in colour as a result of increased vascularity. The vulval veins may become varicose.

The Fallopian Tubes

These are lifted up out of the pelvis as the uterus grows, and at term they are nearly vertical in position. A decidual reaction, similar to that of the uterus but much smaller in degree, occurs in the mucous membrane lining the tubes.

The Ovaries

The ovaries are raised out of the pelvis as the uterus enlarges and at term come to lie just below the costal margins. As a result of stimulation by the chorionic gonadotrophin excreted by the embedding blastocyst, the corpus luteum becomes greatly enlarged during early pregnancy, as described in Chapter 5. At the twelfth week of pregnancy when it has reached its maximum size, it is a yellow body, about ¾ inch (19 mm.) in diameter, containing a small cystic cavity. When seen under the microscope, its cells (luteal cells) are seen to be highly active, containing colloid particles and globules of secretion. It is known as the corpus luteum of pregnancy.

The function of the corpus luteum is to produce oestrogens and progesterone, whose actions have been described in Chapter 4.

After the third month the corpus luteum retrogresses; it becomes much smaller in size, hyaline material is deposited within it and its hormonal activity is greatly reduced. The placenta now takes over its hormone-secreting function which it maintains until the end of pregnancy. Even so, the corpus luteum retains some activity until this time, but after labour it shrinks still further and becomes converted into a corpus albicans.

FURTHER CHANGES IN THE ABDOMEN

The Alimentary Tract

The growing uterus displaces the alimentary tract, and the stomach and intestines become packed away beneath the ribs and in the flanks. The appendix is raised up out of the iliac fossa and is situated below the right costal margin at term.

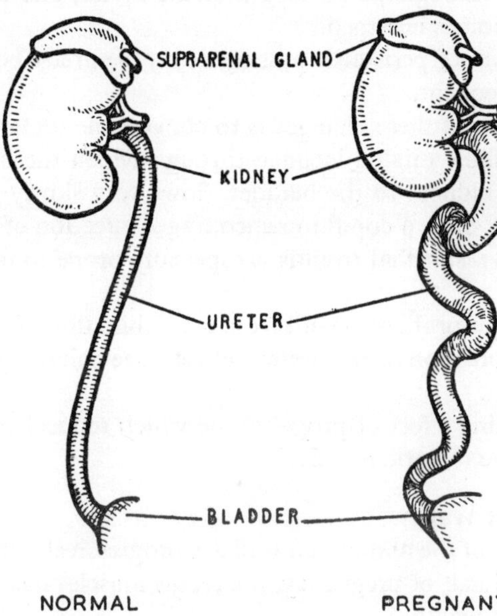

FIGURE 81. Diagram showing the changes in the ureter during pregnancy

The Urinary System

The bladder remains a pelvic organ during pregnancy, but in some patients if the foetal head becomes engaged during the ninth month, the bladder is then displaced into the lower abdomen. This happens more frequently however when the patient goes into labour.

Increased frequency of micturition may be caused in early pregnancy by the weight of the anteverted pregnant uterus, and, following engagement of the head in late pregnancy, by the pressure of the presenting part.

Marked changes occur in the ureters during pregnancy, particularly in primigravidae and on the right side. They occur from the third month onwards, and chiefly affect the part of the ureter lying above the pelvic brim. These changes are as follows:

(i) The affected part of the ureter becomes dilated and elongated.

(ii) The increased length leads to the development of curves and kinks.

(iii) The kinks partially obstruct the flow of urine, so that dilated lacunae occur throughout the length of the ureter, and the pelvis of the kidney becomes enlarged.

(iv) The waves of peristalsis passing down the ureter become slow, weak and infrequent.

The net result of these changes is to convert the ureter into a succession of shallow dilated lacunae through which the urine, on its way from the kidneys to the bladder, flows very slowly and is relatively stagnant. Such a condition encourages infection of the urinary tract, with the result that pyelitis is especially prone to occur during pregnancy.

These changes probably result from a combination of two factors:

1. The compression of the ureter between the enlarging uterus and the pelvic brim.

2. The relaxing effect of progesterone which reduces the tone and efficiency of the ureteric muscle.

The Abdominal Wall

The muscles of the abdominal wall are progressively stretched during the second half of pregnancy, the rectus muscles increasing some three inches in length.

Pinkish streaks known as lineae or striae gravidarum make their appearance in the skin of the abdomen, breasts, buttocks, and upper part of the thighs as pregnancy advances. They were originally thought to be due to rupture of the yellow elastic fibres of the skin brought about by stretching; they are now considered to result from altered function of the suprarenal glands during pregnancy. After delivery they remain permanently present as silvery white scars.

Pigment becomes deposited in the linea alba in some patients, producing what is known as the linea nigra (see p. 161).

CHANGES IN THE BREASTS

Changes in the breasts are described in Chapter 9.

PIGMENTARY CHANGES

Pigmentation of the skin frequently occurs during pregnancy and is thought to be due to a hormone known as melanocyte stimulating hormone (MSH), which comes from the posterior part of the anterior lobe of the pituitary gland and perhaps from the placenta. It stimulates increased growth of pigment cells in the affected areas of skin to cause the characteristic pigmentation. It is more marked in brunettes than in blondes. The chief sites affected are:

1. *The breasts.* The area of pink skin surrounding the nipple in the nullipara changes about the twelfth week of pregnancy into a zone of brownish discoloration. It is known as the primary areola of pregnancy and persists for the remainder of the woman's life.

Surrounding the primary areola an additional wide zone of pigmentation occurs in some women about the 24th week of pregnancy. It forms a dappled mosaic pattern, and is said to resemble raindrops on a plate of mud; it is known as the secondary areola of pregnancy. It disappears after delivery and lactation.

2. *The face.* A golden-brown pigmentation may develop on the face of some women during pregnancy. It is known as chloasma uterinum. It disappears after delivery.

3. *The linea alba.* Brown pigment may become deposited along the linea alba extending from the mons veneris to the umbilicus, so converting it into the linea nigra. Sometimes an area of pigment develops around the umbilicus and the line extends up into the epigastrium. This pigmentation slowly disappears after delivery.

4. *The vulva.* The labia minora become pigmented during pregnancy.

5. *Scars.* A brown pigment may also be deposited in laparotomy scars at this time.

CHANGES IN OTHER SYSTEMS

Circulatory System

The Blood

The total maternal blood volume becomes greater during pregnancy, beginning about the twelfth week and reaching a maximum increase of 25 per cent by the thirtieth week and decreasing slightly thereafter until term. There is a smaller increase in the number of red cells (about 13 per cent) and the haemoglobin (8 per cent) so that a relative dilution of the blood occurs. This is known as hydraemic plethora and produces what is called a physiological anaemia of pregnancy. It is now thought, however, that this anaemia is not physiological in character, but is instead a consequence of iron deficiency. The white cells increase during pregnancy up to 12,000 per c.mm. and may reach 30,000 per c.mm. twelve hours after labour. The platelets are more numerous during pregnancy, and at term amount to 500,000 per c.mm. A typical blood count during pregnancy is:

Erythrocytes	4,000,000 per c.mm.
Haemoglobin	85 per cent
White blood cells	12,000 per c.mm.
Platelets	500,000 per c.mm.

The plasma proteins are reduced, the albumin more than the globulin, and a similar reduction occurs in the alkali reserve, the non-protein nitrogen, blood urea and blood uric acid. The blood calcium falls slightly. There are slight increases in the blood levels of inorganic phosphorus, fibrinogen, lipoids and cholesterol. The blood amino-acids and glucose remain normal whilst the pH remains constant at 7·40.

The Heart

The heart has increased work to perform during pregnancy and so undergoes slight hypertrophy. It is displaced during the later months of pregnancy, being raised and slightly rotated by the rising fundus of the uterus.

The Blood-pressure

The blood-pressure remains normal in pregnancy, and should at no time exceed 130/80 mm. Hg. A slight fall commonly occurs during the middle trimester.

The Veins

The veins of the legs, rectum, anal canal and vulva may become varicose during pregnancy. This is due partly to the pressure of the enlarging uterus, and partly to the relaxing effect which progesterone exerts on the muscle in the vein walls. The chief venous drainage of the pregnant uterus is by way of the ovarian veins, but there is also an increased return through the internal iliac veins. It is thought that this increased flow dams back the venous return from the legs and vulva in the external iliac veins at the point where the veins unite; this raises the pressure in the external iliac veins and so encourages varicosities to develop in their peripheral branches. Constipation predisposes to the production of haemorrhoids.

Respiratory System

The lung bases are compressed by the rising uterine fundus during late pregnancy, and respiration becomes more costal in type; the volume of tidal air which enters and leaves the lungs during normal respiration becomes slightly increased. The vital capacity does not change as pregnancy advances.

Alimentary System

Nausea and morning sickness occur during the first three months in about 50 per cent of all pregnant women. A capricious appetite sometimes develops during the first four months and the patient may have a craving for fruit, vegetables, confectionery, etc.; rarely a liking may appear for unusual substances such as coal, soap and toothpaste. This latter phenomenon is known as pica.

Nervous System

Many women become nervous and irritable during pregnancy.

Skeletal System

The bones and teeth are unchanged during normal pregnancy.

The joints show an increased range of movement, due to the relaxing effect of relaxin on the joint ligaments. This includes the relaxation of the pelvic joints which takes place during labour.

Endocrine System

Many of the ductless glands of the body undergo changes during pregnancy, as follows:

(i) *The pituitary gland.* The anterior lobe swells in size, and large cells, known as pregnancy cells, make their appearance.

The posterior lobe remains unchanged throughout pregnancy although there is an increased production of anti-diuretic hormone (ADH) in cases of pre-eclamptic toxaemia and eclampsia.

(ii) *The suprarenal glands.* No changes occur in the medulla.

The cortex becomes hypertrophied and the production of steroid hormones is increased. It is thought that oestrogens and progesterone are elaborated here during pregnancy.

(iii) *The thyroid gland.* This enlarges during pregnancy, probably in association with the increased metabolic rate.

(iv) *The ovaries.* The function of these glands during pregnancy has already been described.

(v) *The placenta.* This functions as an endocrine organ during pregnancy, as described in Chapter 6.

HORMONAL CHANGES DURING PREGNANCY

1. *Oestrogens.* The amount of oestrogens in the body increases steadily throughout pregnancy, being derived from the corpus luteum during the first three months and from the placenta during the last six. They are also made by the cortex of the suprarenal glands. They are present in free or active forms, but are excreted in combined or inactive states, and probably play a part in initiating the strong uterine contractions of labour.

The three main types of oestrogen present during pregnancy are oestradiol, oestrone and oestriol. Oestriol is found in the largest quantity during pregnancy.

2. *Progesterone.* This increases steadily in quantity throughout pregnancy, also being produced from the corpus luteum during the first three months and from the placenta during the final six months, and from the suprarenal cortex. Its production falls just before the onset of labour, for which it may be partly responsible. It is excreted in the form of pregnanediol.

3. *Chorionic gonadotrophin.* This is produced from the time the blastocyst begins to embed. It rises to a maximum during the second month of pregnancy and then falls, although it is still present until after delivery or death of the placenta occurs.

4. *Relaxin.* This non-steroid hormone is also present during pregnancy, as described in Chapter 6.

5. *Suprarenal steroid hormones.* The increased suprarenal steroid hormones (mineralocorticoids and glucocorticoids) probably come partly from the suprarenal glands and partly from the placenta. Adrenocorticotrophin (ACTH) may also be made by the placenta during pregnancy.

CHANGES IN METABOLISM

During pregnancy the patient needs a diet sufficient to provide 2,800 calories daily. After the fifth month the basal metabolic rate increases, and her weight rises steadily so that by term she has usually gained between 20 to 30 lb. (9 to 13·6 kilograms). This additional weight is made up as follows:

	lb.	Kilos.
The foetus	7	3·2
The placenta	1	0·5
The liquor amnii	3	1·4
The enlarged uterus	2	0·9
The enlarged breasts	2	0·9
Retained body fluids in the blood and tissues generally	5 to 15	2·3 to 6·8
Total	20 to 30	9·2 to 13·7

Although the weight gain averages about ½ lb. (0·23 kg.) per week throughout pregnancy, there is a marked variation in individual patients and at different times in pregnancy. It has been shown that normal pregnant patients gain about 2·5 lb. (1·1 kg.) during the first 12 weeks, 0·92 lb. (0·42 kg.) per week between the 13th and 20th weeks, 1·03 lb. (0·47 kg.) per week between the 20th and 30th weeks, and 0·87 lb. (0·40 kg.) per week thereafter, making a total gain of about 27 lb. (12·2 kg.). Many patients, however, have weight gains that differ widely from these figures, and apart from the presence of twins, hydramnios and oedema due to incidental medical causes, or the deposition of fat, these variations may be ascribed to different amounts of fluid that are retained in the tissues. It is known that the larger the weight gain, and hence the more fluid retained, the greater is the likelihood that the patient may develop pre-eclampsia and eclampsia; thus in one group of patients gaining 1·75 lb (0·79 kg.) or more per week between the 20th and 36th weeks the incidence of pre-eclampsia was 26·0 per cent, whilst amongst those gaining an average of 0·5 lb. (0·23 kg.) or less per week it was only 2·6 per cent.

Some prognostic value may be attached to the amount of weight gained during pregnancy. Thus it is stated that the great majority of patients who gain less than 8 lb. (3·6 kg.) between the 20th and 30th weeks or any earlier 10-week period, will not develop pre-eclampsia later.

When frank oedema develops, whether due to pre-eclamptic toxaemia or any other cause, the weight gain may greatly exceed the figures quoted.

Conversely a small weight gain during pregnancy may be due to excessive vomiting or an incidental disease, and is sometimes associated with impaired growth of the foetus and premature delivery. An actual loss of weight may be due to the same causes, or may precede or follow foetal death in utero.

Fluid Balance

The intake and output of water are both capable of measurement, and for normal health to be maintained a balance should be kept between them. Thus water is taken by mouth, is contained in the solid food eaten, and is produced as the end product of metabolic processes in the body. The excretion of water takes place in the urine, in the faeces, by expiration from the lungs, and by perspiration from the skin. The approximate daily fluid balance may be stated to be:

Intake		*Output*	
By mouth	1,500	Urine	1,500
In solid food	800	Faeces	100
From metabolic processes	300	Respiration	400
		Perspiration	600
Total	2,600 ml.		2,600 ml.

These figures are of course subject to wide variation according to the activity of the patient, the temperature of her surroundings, and many other factors.

The water balance is intimately connected with the levels of electrolytes in the blood, in the tissues, and in the cells themselves. Thus common salt, which produces sodium ions and chloride ions in the body fluids, retains water in the tissues to the extent of 1 litre for every 7 grams of salt. If it is present in excess it will cause fluid retention amounting to oedema, and so diminish the urinary output.

In some diseases, however, the fluid balance may be greatly upset, in which event the measurement of the patient's fluid intake and output and salt balance becomes important. Thus if there is an increased fluid loss by vomiting or diarrhoea the intake should be correspondingly increased either by mouth or by the parenteral route, otherwise dehydration and ketosis may follow. If the amount of salt in the body is reduced, shown by the absence of excreted chlorides in the urine, or diminished sodium and chloride ions (electrolytes) in the plasma, salt should also be given by these routes. Conversely, if the output is decreased and the intake remains unchanged, fluid will be retained in the tissues, excessive weight gain will occur and oedema may appear. This may also occur if excess salt is taken by the patient. Water, however, should not be denied an oedematous patient, for in this event there is insufficient fluid to allow the kidneys to excrete the salt already present, with the result that water is sucked out of the body cells as an alternative source of supply with consequent harmful effects.

The measurement of the fluid intake and output in pre-eclampsia is important, as oliguria signifies increasing fluid retention, worsening of the oedema and possibly the supervention of eclampsia. In cases of anuria, the fluid intake should be correspondingly reduced, only sufficient fluid being supplied to compensate for the water lost by vomiting, respiration and perspiration; the amount of the plasma electrolytes, calcium, potassium and bicarbonate, in addition to sodium and chloride ions, should also be estimated, and they must be maintained at normal levels by the appropriate oral or intravenous therapy.

Metabolism of Proteins

There is a positive retention of nitrogen in the body during pregnancy, which is necessary to build up the tissues of the foetus and the placenta, in addition to the maternal organs which enlarge during this time. About 300 grammes of nitrogen are stored in the body between the 24th week of pregnancy and term. Owing to the diluted state of the blood, the quantitative estimation of blood proteins (albumen and globulin) yields results lower than normal, but, as a result of the increased blood volume, their total amount in the body is increased.

The blood urea during pregnancy is low (7 to 15 mg. per cent) due to this conservation of protein.

Metabolism of Carbohydrates

An adequate intake of carbohydrate in the diet is essential to the pregnant woman, for if it is insufficient, or if she loses carbohydrates by vomiting, ketone bodies appear in the blood and urine very rapidly.

During the process of digestion, carbohydrates are broken down into glucose in the intestine in the usual way, and are absorbed into the blood in this form. Many pregnant women excrete glucose in the urine, as a result of the following abnormalities of carbohydrate metabolism:

1. Renal Glycosuria

In this condition the tubules of the kidney are unable to re-absorb the normal amount of glucose which passes through the glomeruli of the kidney into the urine, and the patient consequently has glycosuria. It is quite independent of the level of the blood sugar, which may in fact be quite low. It is diagnosed from the appearance of the blood-sugar curve, and it needs no treatment. It usually resolves after delivery.

2. Alimentary Glycosuria

When this occurs glucose is absorbed from the intestine into the blood more quickly than it can be stored in the liver. The result is that the amount of glucose in the blood becomes greatly increased after a meal, more passes through the glomeruli than the tubules can re-absorb, and so glycosuria results. This is diagnosed from the blood-sugar curve, which temporarily reaches a high level after the intake of food, but falls to normal within a period of two hours. This condition usually clears up after delivery, though sometimes true diabetes mellitus follows later. No treatment is required during pregnancy.

3. True Diabetes Mellitus

This sometimes complicates pregnancy. The patient may have symptoms of diabetes (thirst, polyuria, polydipsia, constipation), and the blood-sugar rises to a high level which is maintained for longer than two hours. Careful treatment and management of these patients during pregnancy and labour are essential.

Lactose may also occur in the urine of pregnant women, though it is more frequent during lactation. It may be differentiated from glucose by dipping a reagent strip containing a specific enzyme which attacks glucose but not lactose into the urine to be tested. If glucose is present, hydrogen peroxide is formed and this is acted upon by another enzyme present to produce a purple colour; in the presence of lactose, or any other sugar, the reagent strip remains unchanged.

Lactosuria calls for no treatment.

Metabolism of Fats

The metabolism of fats occurs normally in the pregnant woman, although the amount of fat in the blood is increased during pregnancy. Fats are broken down in the tissues into ketone bodies which are used to produce energy. In the absence of sufficient carbohydrates to satisfy energy requirements, an excessive amount of ketone bodies is produced which then appear in the urine (where they are recognized by Acetest tablets or Rothera's test), and constitute a state of ketosis. The pregnant woman develops ketosis in this way much more rapidly than does a woman who is not pregnant.

Metabolism of Minerals

(a) *Iron.* It has already been pointed out that the baby's body contains about 400 mg. of iron at the time of birth, and that the maternal haemoglobin increases by about 8 per cent during pregnancy. Altogether it has been calculated that the mother requires about 900 mg. of additional iron during this time if a state of anaemia is to be avoided. It is true that iron is not lost by menstruation during pregnancy, but this loss amounts to no more than a total of 250 mg. About 20 mg. of iron per day have to be absorbed by the mother to make up the deficiency, and this amount may be obtained from her diet and from iron supplements. A good mixed daily diet of lean meat, liver, eggs, dried fruits, and green leaf vegetables contains only about 15 mg. of iron, of which only 3 to 4 mg. are absorbed by the patient, even when she is suffering from iron-deficiency anaemia. This is because iron passes with difficulty through the intestinal mucosa. Iron supplements, therefore, are very frequently prescribed during pregnancy. It has been found that ferrous salts are better absorbed than ferric salts, and that their absorption is promoted by the presence of hydrochloric acid in the gastric juice and by ascorbic acid. Supplementary iron is therefore usually given as ferrous sulphate tablets in a dosage of 400 mg. per day, of which only 20 mg. or so are absorbed. This compound, however, gives rise to gastric disturbances in about 20 per cent of pregnant women, in which case ferrous gluconate (900 mg.) or ferrous succinate (450 mg.) is substituted for it. Sometimes folic acid (0·5 to 1·7 mg.) is incorporated into the iron tablets, with the result that both forms of anaemia, iron-deficiency anaemia and megaloblastic folic acid deficiency anaemia, are prevented during pregnancy.

Owing to these difficulties with iron absorption it is sometimes given intravenously in the form of saccharated iron oxide containing 20 mg. of iron per ml. of solution, or an iron-dextran complex containing 50 mg. per ml. may be given by the intramuscular route. A total dose infusion of iron in the form of the iron-dextran complex may be given. In this case the amount of iron required to raise the haemoglobin level to normal is calculated and the required dose in normal saline or 5 per cent dextrose is given at one time by a slow intravenous drip, careful attention being paid to ensure that the patient has no adverse reaction. The iron enters the body stores and is converted into haemoglobin during the following weeks and the state of anaemia is abolished.

(b) *Calcium.* This mineral is required for adequate formation of the foetal bones and tooth follicles, and in preparation for future lactation. A daily intake of 1·7 grammes is required. This may be obtained from milk, oatmeal, fruit and vegetables in the diet.

(c) *Phosphorus.* This is also required for bone and tooth follicle formation. About 2 grammes of phosphorus are needed daily and are provided by milk, cheese, egg yolk, lean meat and vegetables in the diet.

(d) *Iodine.* This is necessary because the mother's basal metabolic rate is raised during pregnancy, and this is dependent upon an increased secretion of the thyroid hormone, thyroxin. The foetus also requires a small amount of iodine. A daily intake of 0·1 mg. is sufficient, obtained by eating sea-fish or fish-liver oil twice weekly.

CHAPTER 9

The Anatomy and Physiology of the Breasts

THE ANATOMY OF THE BREASTS

The female breasts consist of two hemispherical swellings situated in the superficial fascia of the anterior chest wall. Over the centre of each breast there is a circular area, about one inch (2·5 cm.) in diameter, known as the areola, which is coloured pink in nulliparae and brownish in women who have borne children. In the centre of the areola is placed the nipple, a flat-topped papillary protuberance about ¼ inch (6 mm.) in length. In nulliparae it points forwards and slightly outwards and upwards, whilst in women who have borne children and lactated, it lies at a lower level and may point downwards.

The breast extends from the second rib above to the sixth rib below, medially it reaches the lateral margin of the sternum, whilst laterally it extends as far as the mid-axillary line. Its circular shape is not complete, as part of the breast from the upper and outer quadrant extends up into the axilla, reaching as high as the third rib. This is known as the axillary tail of Spence.

The breast lies mainly over the pectoralis major muscle, though it partly overlaps the serratus anterior and the external oblique muscles.

The nipple of the nullipara is situated about the level of the fourth intercostal space, and is pink in colour. Its surface is perforated by fifteen to twenty minute orifices which are the openings of the lactiferous tubules. Within the areola are situated about 18 sebaceous glands, which become enlarged into tubercles during pregnancy.

Structure

The substance of the breast is composed of glandular tissue which is gathered into about 18 lobes. These lobes radiate outwards from the areola in the manner of spokes in a wheel, and they are separated

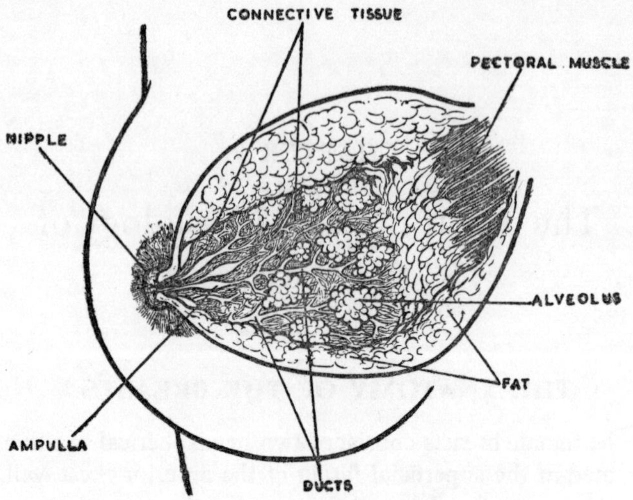

FIGURE 82. Dissection of breast to show its structure

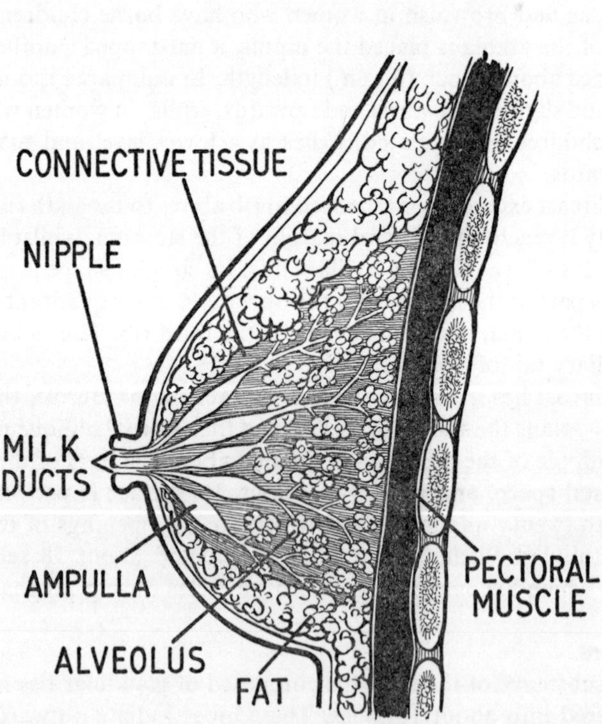

FIGURE 83. Section through breast to show its attachment to the chest wall

from each other, within the breast, by fibrous connective tissue partitions. Each lobe is thus a complete unit and lies next to, but does not communicate with, its fellows.

Each of the 18 lobes is divided by smaller partitions into numerous lobules, which are made up of masses of milk-excreting units known as alveoli. Each alveolus consists of a number of milk-forming cells surrounding a small duct into which they pour their excretion. During pregnancy this takes the form of colostrum, but after delivery it becomes changed to milk. The ducts from the alveoli join together and form larger ducts; these unite with ducts from other lobules, until finally a large duct, known as a lactiferous tubule, emerges from the entire lobe and runs towards the nipple.

Whilst it passes beneath the areola, each lactiferous tubule expands and forms a dilated sac known as an ampulla, which serves as a reservoir for milk. From here the tubule from each lobe enters the nipple and opens independently upon its surface.

The walls of the ducts are lined by a layer of cubical cells which rest upon a basement membrane and are surrounded by a cellular connective tissue. The larger ducts near the nipple are enclosed by smooth muscle cells. The alveoli and the smaller ducts are surrounded by spider-shaped contractile cells known as myo-epithelial or basket cells.

The gland is stabilized in the fat of the chest wall by numerous fibrous processes which pass from the gland tissue to the skin, areola and subcutaneous tissues, forming a fibrous investment to the whole gland. These are known as the ligaments of Astley-Cooper.

Blood Supply

The breast is supplied with blood by:

(i) The internal mammary artery, which is a branch of the subclavian artery coming from the innominate artery on the right and the aorta on the left.

(ii) The external mammary artery, which is derived from the lateral thoracic artery, a branch of the axillary artery which is the continuation of the subclavian artery.

(iii) The upper intercostal arteries, which pass along the intercostal spaces deep to the breast, coming mainly from the aorta.

The veins form a circular network around the nipple and drain to the internal mammary and axillary veins.

Lymph Drainage

The lymph vessels form a plexus beneath the areola and between the lobes of the breast. The lymphatics of the two breasts communicate freely with each other.

The lymph drains to the following regional nodes:

(i) The axillary glands in both axillae.
(ii) The glands in the anterior mediastinum.
(iii) The glands in the portal fissure of the liver.

Nerve Supply

The functioning of the breast is controlled by hormones, and it has a poor nerve supply. Some sympathetic fibres pass to it with the blood-vessels; the skin over the breast is supplied by cutaneous branches of the fourth, fifth and sixth thoracic nerves.

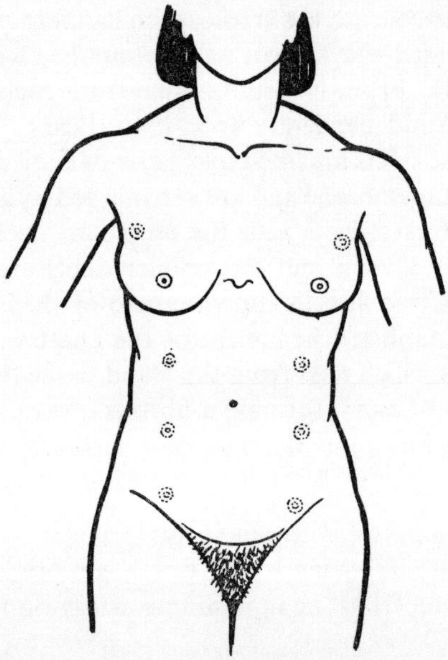

FIGURE 84. Diagram showing positions of accessory nipples

Accessory Breasts

In the early foetal life of all mammals a line of immature breasts extends from the axilla to the inguinal region on each side. The majority of these breasts disappear, the number of those persisting being related to the size of the litter the animal will later produce; in the human race all normally disappear except two which develop into the adult structures described above. Sometimes, however, small breasts and nipples persist along this line, which are known as accessory breasts and nipples. These undergo pregnancy changes and actually excrete milk during the puerperium, rarely in fact rivalling the proper breasts in size and function. Usually, however, they are small, and the patient often mistakes them for pigmented moles.

BREAST CHANGES DURING PREGNANCY

Examination of the breasts during pregnancy reveals changes which begin about the sixth week. These are as follows:

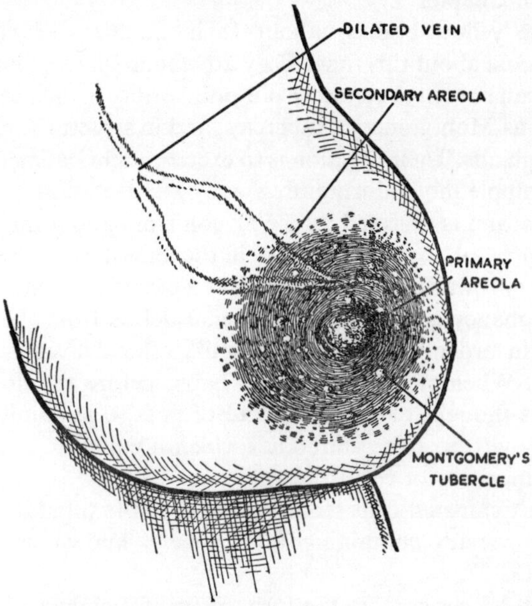

FIGURE 85. Drawing of the pregnant breast

(i) The structure of the breast tissue becomes changed from a soft smooth texture to one which is nodular and lumpy to the feel. This is first detected at the periphery of the breast and is due to the growth and enlargement of the alveoli of the breast parenchyma. The alveoli are in fact growing in response to stimulation by progesterone, in preparation for the future excretion of milk after delivery. As this growth continues during pregnancy, the whole breast gradually becomes larger in size.

(ii) An increased vascularity of the breast occurs. This is seen under the skin of the breasts as a plexiform network of subcutaneous veins. As pregnancy advances it becomes more intricate and widespread, until at term the veins ramify over the whole anterior aspect of the thorax. This venous network can be detected by infra-red photography from the time of the first missed period, a fact which may be employed in making the diagnosis of early pregnancy.

About the twelfth week of pregnancy further changes occur:

(iii) The nipple becomes more prominent, and the areola develops an increased fullness and pigmentation. Its pink colour changes to a brownish hue, forming the primary areola of pregnancy. This is described in Chapter 8.

(iv) Some yellow bodies—about 18 in number—develop in the primary areola about this time. They are about $\frac{1}{8}$ inch (3 mm.) in diameter and can be seen to contain a pin-point orifice in their centre. They are known as Montgomery's tubercles, and in structure are modified sebaceous glands. Their function is to excrete a lubricating fluid which keeps the nipple moist during pregnancy and lactation.

(v) Colostrum is excreted by the alveoli from about this time, and can be expressed from the nipple if the breast is massaged from the periphery towards the centre. This is a clear fluid, whose function during pregnancy is to remove epithelial debris from the lumen of the ducts, in order that the flow of milk after delivery will not be obstructed. When swallowed by the baby, before the flow of milk begins, it is thought to confer a state of passive immunity to some diseases, by virtue of the antibodies which it contains.

The composition of colostrum is:

(a) Desquamated cells from the walls of the tubules.

(b) Leucocytes containing fat droplets, known as colostrum corpuscles.

(c) Fat 2·5 per cent, in the form of free fat globules.

(d) About 8 per cent protein, in the forms of lactalbumen and lactoglobulin.

(e) Lactose 3·5 per cent.

(f) Inorganic salts.

Colostrum is alkaline in reaction with a calorie value of 21 calories per ounce.

(vi) About the 24th week of pregnancy a secondary areola sometimes appears, most often in brunettes. It has already been described in Chapter 8.

These changes are physiologically the body's preparation for subsequent lactation, but they may be used clinically to diagnose the presence of pregnancy. Sometimes however they are unreliable diagnostic criteria; thus they may be only slightly developed when pregnancy is well advanced, whilst conversely they may appear to a marked degree in patients who are not pregnant, but who have instead a hormone-bearing ovarian tumour or uterine fibroids. In some cases the changes are induced by psychological states.

THE PHYSIOLOGY OF THE BREASTS

The later development of the breasts begins at the time of puberty, but they cannot be said to attain full maturity until the patient becomes a lactating mother.

At puberty the breasts enlarge and assume the adult female size and shape. This is in response to stimulation by oestrogens, which reach the breasts through the blood stream from the growing Graafian follicles. Oestrogens cause a certain amount of growth of the nipple and areola, but their main function at this time is to promote growth and development of the lactiferous tubules and ducts. The breast enlargement at puberty, therefore, is due to the expansion of the duct system of the breast, under oestrogenic influence.

Non-pregnant patients sometimes complain of fullness and tinglings of the breasts before a menstrual period. This is thought to be due to congestion occurring at this time, as a result of stimulation by progesterone derived from the corpus luteum of menstruation.

Further development and enlargement of the breasts next occur during pregnancy. The most important feature at this time is the hypertrophy of the alveoli in response to progesterone stimulation, preparatory to the later manufacture of milk. As the whole breast hypertrophies during pregnancy, new glandular tissue with its ducts develops, and both hormones, oestrogens and progesterone, play their respective parts in this process.

About the third day after delivery milk appears in the breasts as a result of stimulation by prolactin derived from the acidophil cells of the anterior pituitary, and they can then be said to have reached their full development.

THE COMPOSITION OF MILK

The composition of human milk is variable, but the average percentages of its constituents are as follows:

	Per cent
1. Proteins	1·5
(Caseinogen 0·5 per cent Lactalbumen 1·0 per cent)	
2. Lactose	7·0
3. Fat	3·5
4. Salts	0·2
(Phosphates and chlorides of calcium, sodium and potassium)	
5. Water	87·8
Total	100·0

Milk is alkaline in reaction (pH 7·0 to 7·6), has a specific gravity of 1031 and a caloric value of 20 calories per ounce.

THE PHYSIOLOGY OF LACTATION

The process of lactation can be considered to take place in 3 stages:

1. The actual production of milk in the alveoli.
2. The flow of milk along the ducts to the nipple.
3. The withdrawal of milk from the nipple by the baby.

1. The Production of Milk

Milk is formed as small fatty globules within the cytoplasm of the cells of the alveoli. The globules arise in the bases of these cells, and gradually unite to form small droplets. As new globules are produced the droplets are pushed towards the surface of the cell until finally they burst through the cell membrane and enter the lactiferous tubule, accompanied by a little cytoplasm of the cell substance. Here they join with droplets from other cells and the terminal portions of the tubules within the excreting alveoli become filled with milk.

Breasts which excrete milk in this way require a large blood supply and it has been calculated that milk is formed from a volume of blood about 350 times greater than that of the milk produced. The composition of milk is dependent on the metabolism of the alveolar cells, which make caseinogen from amino-acids in the blood, and lactose from glucose. The mother's diet does not affect the composition of milk, with the exception of fat, which may change its constitution if large quantities of different kinds of fat are taken in the diet.

The manufacture of milk is under the control of the hormone prolactin, which is derived from the anterior lobe of the pituitary gland. The action of the hormone is suppressed by oestrogens, and it is not until a few days after the expulsion of the placenta that the amount of oestrogens in the blood is sufficiently reduced to allow prolactin to exert its influence on the alveolar cells and so lead to milk production. It is then recognised clinically that 'the milk comes in' about the third day of the puerperium. Once lactation has been established by prolactin, growth hormone, which comes also from the anterior pituitary, appears to play some part in its maintenance.

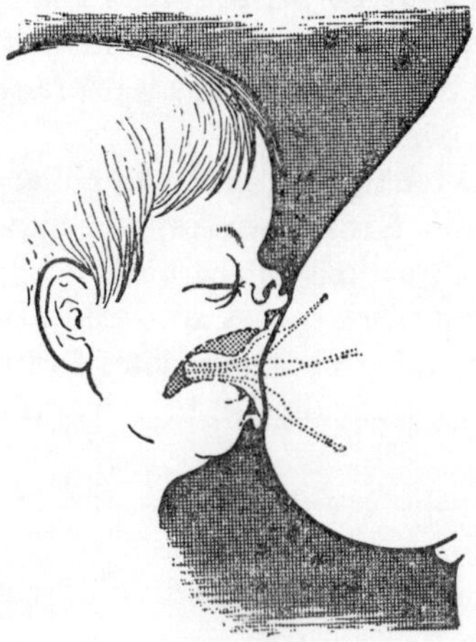

FIGURE 86.
Drawing showing the positions of the nipple and ampullae during feeding

2. The Flow of Milk

The milk is pushed along the ducts towards the nipple by the milk which is being continually formed behind it in the alveoli. Some of the milk is stored in the ampullae underneath the areola, until the time of the baby's next feed.

When milk is drawn off by the infant, the smooth muscle and basket cells in the walls of the ducts and alveoli contract and force more milk towards the nipple. This mechanism occurs as a result of a neuro-hormonal reflex. Thus the stimulus of the baby's mouth on the sensitive nipple reaches the brain, and by a nervous reflex a hormone is liberated from the posterior lobe of the pituitary gland. This is known to be oxytocin. It reaches the breast in the blood stream, stimulates the muscle cells and basket cells to contract and causes more milk to flow to the nipple. This gives rise to a sensation, which the mother may feel in both breasts, known as 'the draught'.

The liberated oxytocin may at the same time stimulate the uterus to contract, and it is well recognised clinically that the patient may feel uterine contractions whilst she is feeding her baby.

3. The Withdrawal of Milk

The baby sucks milk from the breasts partly by creating a vacuum in its mouth, but mainly by performing a champing action with its jaws. Thus the baby draws the whole areola and not only the nipple into its mouth, and by closing its jaws it expresses the milk from the ampullae and then swallows it.

As the baby takes the milk from the ampullae and the lower parts of the ducts, more milk flows down from the upper parts of the ducts, propelled by the contractions of the basket cells, until the breast is emptied. The sucking reflex causes an outflow of prolactin from the anterior pituitary gland, which stimulates further milk production. In this way the breast gradually fills in preparation for the next feeding time.

Thus to maintain successful lactation, the necessary requirements are:

(i) An adequate intake of food and fluid by the mother sufficient to provide 3,500 calories per day.

(ii) Well developed breasts and nipples.

(iii) An adequate and frequently repeated sucking stimulus to provide the neuro-hormonal reflexes.

(iv) Complete emptying of the breasts.

(v) A large blood supply to the breasts.

(vi) Ducts freed from epithelial debris.

The provision of these requirements is however outside the realm of physiology, and is part of the clinical technique of successful breast feeding.

APPENDIX I

The Kidneys

ANATOMY

The kidneys are two organs of characteristic shape which lie outside the peritoneum on the posterior abdominal wall, one on each side of the vertebral column. They measure 4 inches in length, $2\frac{1}{2}$ inches in width, and $1\frac{1}{4}$ inches in thickness ($10{\cdot}1 \times 6{\cdot}4 \times 3{\cdot}2$ cm.), and each weighs about 4 ounces (114 grammes). They extend from the upper border of the twelfth thoracic vertebra above, to the third lumbar vetebra below, with the upper pole slightly closer to the middle line than the lower pole. The centre of the inner border is connected by a vascular pedicle with the descending aorta and the inferior vena cava—this lies at the level of the intervertebral disc between the

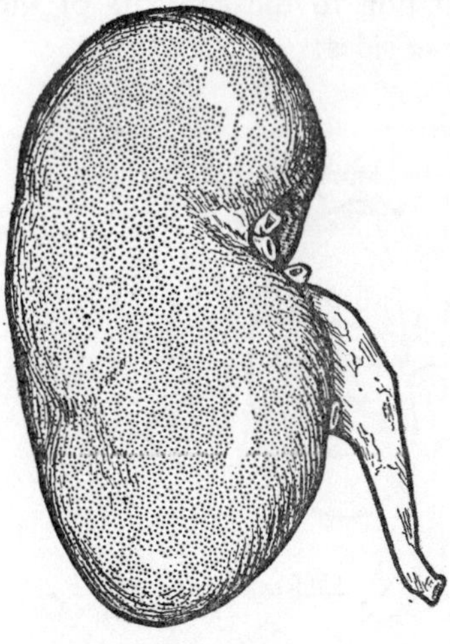

FIGURE 87. Anterior view of a right kidney

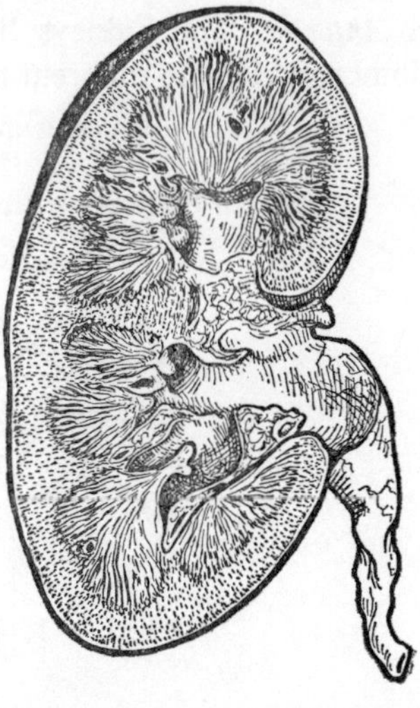

FIGURE 88. A right kidney on section

first and second lumbar vertebrae. The right kidney is placed at a slightly lower level than the left, owing to the presence of the liver in the right hypochondrium.

The kidney is smooth in outline, reddish-brown in colour, with convex surfaces and broadly rounded margins. The upper and lower poles are almost semicircular, whilst the lateral border is gently curved. The medial border is indented in its middle third, a region known as the hilum, where the renal artery enters and the renal vein and ureter leave the kidney. These structures, together with lymphatic vessels and nerves, comprise the renal pedicles. The hilum consists of a cleft lying between thick rounded lips into which these structures pass, the vein, artery and ureter lying in that order from before backwards.

Surface marking

The kidney lies well above the pelvic brim, and is marked on the surface of the abdomen by an area occupying the middle two quarters of the distance between the ensiform cartilage and the umbilicus, its long axis passing downwards and a little outwards, about 3 inches (7·6 cm.) from the middle line.

Relations

1. *Anterior*. The kidneys lie in relation to the contents of the abdomen, which are different on the two sides:

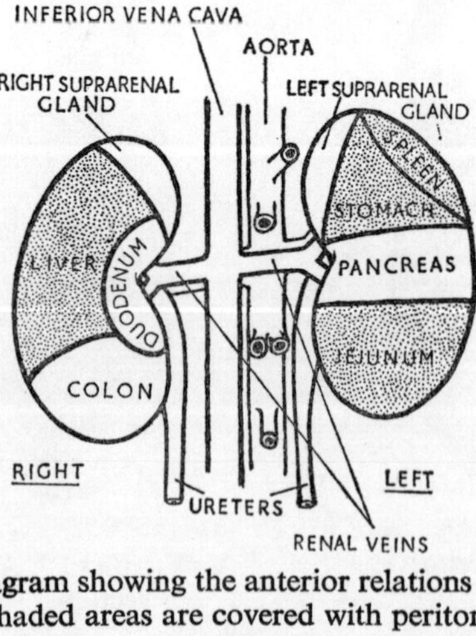

Figure 89. Diagram showing the anterior relations of the kidneys. (The shaded areas are covered with peritoneum)

(*a*) *The left kidney*. The inner aspect of the upper pole is surmounted by the left suprarenal gland, while the outer aspect is related to the spleen. Extending as a horizontal band across the central region lies the pancreas, the triangular area thus demarcated between these organs forming part of the bed of the stomach. The lower pole, below the pancreatic area, lies in relation to the jejunum.

(*b*) *The right kidney*. In a similar manner the inner aspect of the upper pole is related to the right suprarenal gland, whilst the area surrounding the hilum lies behind the duodenum. The liver lies in front of the upper half of the remainder of the anterior surface, whilst the hepatic flexure of the colon is in contact with the lower half.

2. *Posterior*. The kidneys lie in relation to the structures of the posterior abdominal wall, which, apart from the slight lowering of the right kidney, are identical on the two sides.

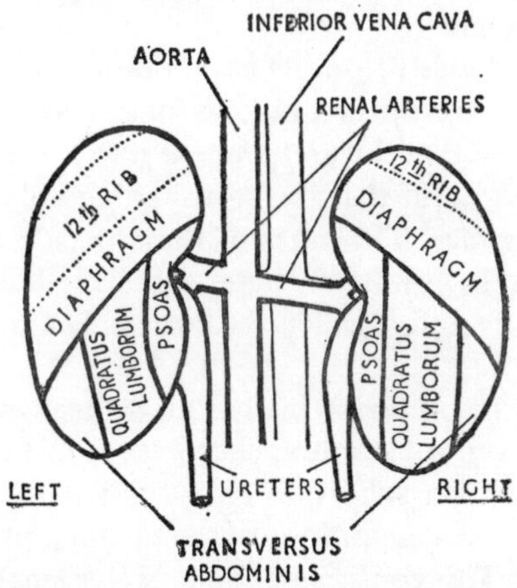

FIGURE 90. Diagram showing the posterior relations of the kidneys. (The pleural cavity lies between the diaphragm and the twelfth rib)

The upper half of each kidney rests against the diaphragm, the twelfth rib passing obliquely outwards and downwards across its surface, but separated from it by the diaphragmatic muscle fibres. Between the diaphragm and the rib the pleural cavity is a posterior relation, especially on the left side where the kidney is higher.

The lower half of the kidney lies against three muscles of the posterior abdominal wall, which, passing outwards from the spine, are the psoas major, the quadratus lumborum, and the transversus abdominis.

Supports

The kidney is closely covered by a thick fibrous capsule, and lies embedded in loose cellular tissue containing copious deposits of fat, known as the perinephric fat. It is supported in this position by:

(i) The general intra-abdominal pressure and close contact with adjoining organs.

(ii) The attachment of the renal vessels to the aorta and the inferior vena cava.

(iii) An investment of deep fascia, connected below to the parietal pelvic fascia, which surrounds the kidney. This is attached by fibrous strands to the kidney capsule, and is known in this situation as the renal fascia.

The Kidney on Section

If the kidney is divided from its lateral border towards the hilum, and its two halves are opened out, its naked eye structure can be seen. It will be noted that the ureter opens into a cavity known as the pelvis of the kidney, and that the surrounding kidney substances is divided into two zones. The inner of these is pale in colour and is known as the medulla, whilst the outer zone is reddish brown and of uniform consistency and is called the cortex. The following features are to be noted:

(i) *The pelvis of the kidney.* This has an intimate relation with the medulla. It divides into large branches known as the major calyces, and these in their turn subdivide into smaller branches called the minor calyces, into which portions of the medulla protrude.

(ii) *The medulla.* This consists of about twelve small conical masses which project into the minor calyces of the renal pelvis, with their base extending to about half-way towards the surface. They contain faint parallel streaks which run towards the tip of the projection. These constitute the pyramids of the kidney, whilst the streaks terminating in their apices are known as the medullary rays. These are the collecting tubules which carry urine from the cortex of the kidney to the calyces. From here the urine passes into the pelvis of the kidney and then makes its journey down the ureter into the bladder.

(iii) *The cortex.* This arches over the bases of the pyramids, lying between them and the surface, and in places extends between them to reach to the pelvis. These portions of cortex lying between the pyramids are known as the columns of Bertini.

(iv) *The capsule.* This is a thick fibrous coat which surrounds the cortex, from which it can be stripped. In the body it is attached to the surrounding renal fascia and perinephric fat. Running underneath it external to the cortex lies a series of veins known as the stellate veins.

(v) *The renal blood vessels.* After the renal artery enters the kidney it divides into branches which form arches lying between the cortex and the medulla. These give off small arterioles which enter and supply the cortex. Venous blood is collected into similar arches lying in the boundary between the cortex and medulla, which also receive blood from the stellate veins. They finally unite to form the renal vein.

The Structure of the Kidney

The chief kidney function is to regulate the composition and volume of the blood plasma, which it does by secreting urine, and its structure is designed primarily for this purpose. The urine is produced by about a million small units in each kidney known as nephrons, which are packed closely together in a connecting stroma thereby forming a solid mass which is the kidney substance. It is convenient to study the minute anatomy of one of these structures, the nephron, and its intimate association with the renal blood vessels.

It has already been stated that the renal artery sends branches into the cortex, and as these extend towards the capsule they give off small arterioles which break up into globular clumps of capillaries known as glomeruli. Each of these is invested around its periphery by a thin membrane formed of flat epithelial cells which is reflected back on itself to produce a cup-like structure. The glomerulus thus invaginates the membrane which is called Bowman's capsule. From this capsule a small tubule, known as a uriniferous tubule, arises. The glomerulus, surrounded by Bowman's capsule, forms what is known as a Malpighian body. The vessel carrying blood into the glomerulus is called the afferent arteriole, and the vessel draining blood away from it is the efferent arteriole. Here are therefore two arterioles, one which delivers blood into the glomerular capillaries, and one which drains it away.

After leaving the Malpighian body the uriniferous tubule does not

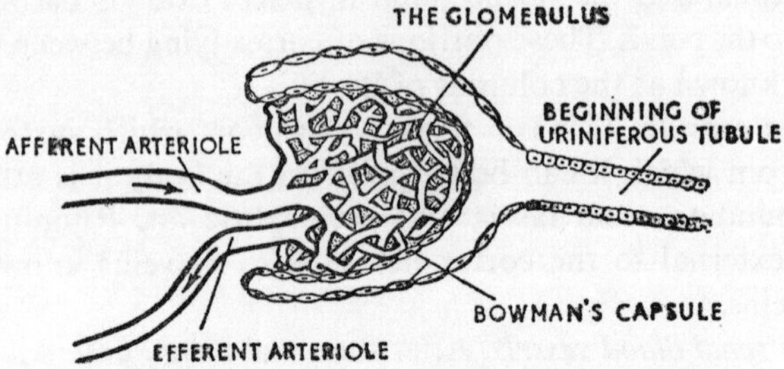

FIGURE 91. Diagram of a Malpighian body

branch, but instead takes a tortuous course, twisting and turning in all directions within the cortex. This part of its course is known as the first convoluted tubule of the nephron. The cubical cells by which it is lined contain particles arranged in parallel rows along the surface. The border of the cells lining the lumen of the tubule thus has a striated appearance which is known as the brush border.

After a series of these convolutions the tubule takes a spiral course, where it is known as the spiral tubule, and then straightens out and dips down into the medulla. It travels a short distance and then makes a U-turn and returns to the cortex. This formation is known as the loop of Henle, and the two limbs of the loop comprise its descending and ascending limbs. The cells lining these limbs differ. Thus the descending limb and the U-bend are lined by flattened cells but have a narrow lumen, whilst the ascending limb contains cubical cells and is much wider.

After returning to the cortex, the tubule takes a crooked course, where it is called the zig-zag tubule, after which a second series of convolutions follows forming the second convoluted tubule. On leaving the convolutions the tubule is called a junctional tubule, which then joins a collecting tubule. This runs from the cortex to the apex of the pyramid, forming the medullary rays which have already been noted, and receiving the terminations of about 4,200 junctional tubules during its course. These are also known as the ducts of Bellini. They open into a minor calyx at the apex of a pyramid, each pyramid containing about twenty ducts.

The efferent arteriole, after leaving the glomerulus, breaks up into a second network of capillaries which surrounds the tubules throughout their course. These ultimately join to form venules, which, uniting with the stellate veins from the capsule, finally form the renal veins.

The original arteriole thus gives rise to two sets of capillaries before the blood joins the vein, one forming the glomerulus and one surrounding the tubules.

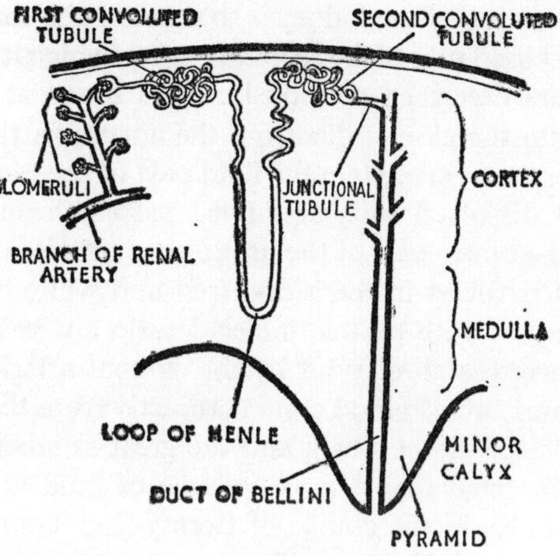

FIGURE 92. Diagram of a nephron

The length of each tubule is about $1\frac{1}{5}$ inches (3 cm.), so that the total length of the tubules of the two million nephrons in the two kidneys is about thirty-eight miles (60 kilometres).

Lymphatic Supply

A plexus of lymph vessels lies beneath the kidney capsule which is connected to a second plexus surrounding the uriniferous tubules. Lymphatic trunks emerge from these plexuses and follow the renal vein to end in the aortic or lumbar lymphatic glands.

Nerve Supply

The kidney is supplied by sympathetic and parasympathetic nerves coming from the renal plexus, which is derived from the coeliac and aortic plexuses and the splanchnic nerves lying on the posterior abdominal wall. Branches accompany the renal artery into the substance of the kidney and are distributed to the blood vessels throughout their ramifications.

The renal plexus sends branches which communicate with the ovarian plexus.

THE KIDNEYS

PHYSIOLOGY

(a) The Formation of Urine

The chief function of the kidney is to regulate the composition and volume of the blood plasma by secreting urine, which it does by virtue of the structure described previously. Thus blood at high pressure is delivered into the glomerulus from the aorta, via the renal artery and the afferent arteriole. Here the fluid part of the blood, consisting of water and dissolved salts and ions, passes through Bowman's capsule into the upper part of the uriniferous tubule. It will be noted that the solid particles in the blood (red and white corpuscles and platelets), together with protein molecules, do not pass through this barrier but leave the glomerulus by the efferent arteriole. Considering the high pressure of blood coming directly from the aorta (about 75 mm. Hg. in the glomerulus), and the great number of nephrons, it would be expected that a large volume of fluid would enter the uriniferous tubules in the course of twenty-four hours—this is certainly true, as some 170 litres (37 gallons) are filtered off from the blood in this way per day.

The fluid (known as the glomerular filtrate) then passes along the whole length of the tubule, and during this journey the greater part of the water, and all the dissolved substances which are of value to the body, are reabsorbed by the cells lining the tubules and are passed back into the circulation. Only waste products of no value to the individual pass on to the collecting tubules and then into the pelvis of the kidney. In this way 168½ litres of fluid are reabsorbed, leaving only 1½ litres to pass down the ureter into the bladder and constitute the urine.

Thus sugar and bicarbonates, and sodium, chloride and calcium ions, are filtered off by the glomeruli but are largely reabsorbed by the tubules; urea, urates, uric acid, sulphates and phosphates which are also filtered off are only reabsorbed to a slight extent and so appear in the urine. The tubular cells thus have the power of reabsorbing substances selectively, according to the body's requirements. Some compounds such as creatinine and ingested toxic substances are excreted by the tubular cells directly into the urine. The function of the tubules therefore is mainly reabsorptive but is partly excretory. The reabsorption takes place chiefly in the ascending limb of the loop of Henle. The reabsorption of water is largely under the control of anti-diuretic hormone, derived from the posterior lobe of the pituitary gland, whilst the reabsorption of sodium ions (which occurs in the second convoluted tubule) is controlled by a hormone known as aldosterone, derived from the suprarenal cortex.

(b) Kidney functions in detail

(i) By this process of urinary formation the kidneys regulate the volume of plasma in the blood and the amount of fluid in the extra-cellular spaces of the tissues. It is well recognized that the more fluid drunk and absorbed, the larger is the volume of urine excreted, whilst if much fluid is lost by perspiration or diarrhoea, the urinary output is reduced.

(ii) The reaction of the blood is kept constant by a similar mechanism. If the hydrogen ion concentration of the blood is increased producing a tendency towards acidity, the ions are excreted in acid urine, in the form of acid phosphate, and the pH of the blood remains constant. Conversely if the hydrogen ion concentration is reduced, alkaline urine, containing alkaline phosphate and possibly bicarbonate, is produced.

(iii) Waste products are excreted in the urine, particularly urea, urates, uric acid, ammonia, creatinine and sulphates, which are all the end-products of protein metabolism.

(iv) Toxic substances introduced into the body are eliminated.

(v) By means of these excretory functions the kidneys regulate the osmotic pressure of the blood and tissue fluids.

(vi) The cortex secretes a hormone known as renin. This is produced when the blood-supply to the kidney is reduced; it combines with a protein called hypertensinogen present in the blood to form a pressor agent, hypertensin or angiotonin, which brings about a rise in blood pressure.

(vii) The kidneys secrete another hormone into the blood stream that stimulates the formation of red blood cells in the marrow. This is known as renal erythropoietin. A reduced secretion, occurring in cases of chronic nephritis, accounts for the anaemia that accompanies this disease.

The kidneys thus have mainly a regulatory and excretory function; they are essential to life and the individual cannot live for long if their function becomes seriously deranged.

APPENDIX II

The Meaning of pH

In describing physiological processes statements are sometimes made such as the 'pH of the blood is 7·40', or 'the pH of the vagina is 4·5'. It is generally understood that these observations indicate the reaction, that is to say the acidity or alkalinity of the substance in question, but in order to appreciate the exact significance of these figures, certain principles of physical chemistry and of mathematics must be borne in mind.

Firstly then it must be understood that compounds are made up of atoms combined together to form molecules. Thus for example common salt (sodium chloride) is composed of an atom of sodium (written Na) combined with an atom of chlorine (written Cl). When such a compound is dissolved in water, the molecules split up, or as it is called 'dissociate', into small electrified particles called ions, those in this case being a sodium ion (written Na^+) which carries a small positive charge of electricity, and a chloride ion (written Cl^-) which carries a small negative charge of electricity. These opposite charges are always equal in number, so that the solution remains electrically balanced. All salts in the body fluids dissociate in this way, so that there are produced potassium ions (K^+), calcium ions (Ca^{++}), sulphate ions (SO_4^{--}), bicarbonate ions (HCO_3^-), etc. (Some ions such as calcium and sulphate carry double charges as shown by the two plus or minus signs.) The ions affect the metabolism of the body, and it is always imperative that they should maintain their normal levels—hence the number of ions must be estimated in ill states such as dehydration, and the correct electrolytic balance must be restored when necessary.

In addition to the ions derived as above water dissociates. A molecule of water is composed of 2 hydrogen atoms combined with 1 oxygen atom, and is written H_2O. It can also be written as H – OH in which case is can be considered to be made up of a hydrogen atom united to an OH group, known as an hydroxyl radicle. When water dissociates it splits up into a hydrogen ion (H^+) and a hydroxyl ion (OH^-). It is these ions that determine the reaction of a solution. Thus if a substance is dissolved in water that makes the hydrogen ions more numerous than the hydroxyl ions the solution will be acid in reaction; if on the other hand the hydroxyl ions outnumber the hydrogen ions, then the solution will be alkaline. This occurs in strict mathematical proportion, i.e., the greater the preponderance of H^+ ions the more acid the solution, and the greater the OH^- ions the more alkaline it becomes. As water itself contains both ions in equal numbers, it is of course neutral in reaction.

When it is necessary to state in figures how acid or alkaline a solution is, numbers have to be employed, and the number chosen relates to the concentrations of hydrogen ions and hydroxyl ions in the solution. We may in fact define the reaction of a solution as being the relative concentrations of hydrogen and hydroxyl ions in that solution. The numbers involved in such statements are very large comprising hundreds, thousands, millions, tens of millions, etc., and these are usually written as powers of ten, so as to avoid writing huge numbers with long rows of noughts. Thus it can be stated that:

10^1 = ten
10^2 = a hundred
10^3 = a thousand
10^4 = ten thousand
10^5 = a hundred thousand
10^6 = a million
10^7 = ten million
10^8 = a hundred million, and so on

In a similar manner:

$$10^{-1} = \frac{1}{10} = \text{one in ten}$$

$$10^{-2} = \frac{1}{100} = \text{one in a hundred}$$

$$10^{-3} = \frac{1}{1{,}000} = \text{one in a thousand}$$

$$10^{-4} = \frac{1}{10{,}000} = \text{one in ten thousand}$$

$$10^{-5} = \frac{1}{100{,}000} = \text{one in a hundred thousand}$$

$$10^{-6} = \frac{1}{1{,}000{,}000} = \text{one in a million}$$

and so on.

Now when water dissociates it only does so to a very small extent. In fact only one molecule in every ten million splits up into hydrogen and hydroxyl ions. The concentration of hydrogen ions is therefore one in every ten million molecules, and this is written:

$$\text{Conc. of H}^+ = \frac{1}{10{,}000{,}000} = \frac{1}{10^7} = 10^{-7}$$

It is this figure 7 which is taken as the basis of pH. Instead of writing the concentration of H^+ ions as above, we simply take the figure 7, ignore the minus sign, and say the pH of water is 7. As mentioned above water is completely neutral in reaction, and it can be said therefore that a pH of 7 represents absolute neutrality.

It is a law in chemistry that when water dissociates in this way, the number of hydrogen ions multiplied by the number of hydroxyl ions always produces a constant number. Thus:

$$\text{Conc. of H}^+ \times \text{Conc. of OH}^- = \text{a constant}$$

$$\frac{1}{10^7} \times \frac{1}{10^7} = \frac{1}{10^{14}}$$

$$10^{-7} \times 10^{-7} = 10^{-14}$$

If therefore the concentration of H^+ ions in water were increased to one in a million $\left(\frac{1}{10^6}\right)$ instead of one in ten millions $\left(\frac{1}{10^7}\right)$, then it would automatically follow that the concentration of hydroxyl ions would decrease, so that the same constant number is obtained when the two concentrations are multiplied together:

H^+ ions		OH^- ions		
10^{-6}	$\times$	10^{-8}	$=$	10^{-14}
10^{-5}	$\times$	10^{-9}	$=$	10^{-14}

and so on. As the concentration of H^+ ions becomes increased the solution becomes more acid and the pH falls as the figure denoting it changes from 7 to 6 to 5, etc.

Similarly if the concentration of hydrogen ions were decreased to one in a hundred million $\left(\frac{1}{10^8}\right)$, then the concentration of hydroxyl ions would increase in a corresponding manner:

H^+ ions		OH^- ions		
10^{-8}	×	10^{-6}	=	10^{-14}
10^{-9}	×	10^{-5}	=	10^{-14}

and so on. As the concentration of H^+ ions becomes less the solution becomes more alkaline and the pH rises as the figure changes from 7 to 8 to 9, etc.

If a substance containing many hydrogen ions such as hydrochloric acid is added to water with a pH of 7, it increases the concentration of hydrogen ions in the water, the hydroxyl ions become progressively fewer and the solution becomes more acid with a pH below 7. If, on the other hand, a substance such as washing soda (sodium carbonate) is added to water it reduces the number of hydrogen ions, with the result that more molecules of water dissociate to maintain the constant number referred to and the hydroxyl ions gradually accumulate and make the solution alkaline, with a pH above 7.

Thus we can say that a solution of hydrochloric acid with a pH of 3 has one hydrogen ion present to every thousand molecules $\left(\frac{1}{10^3}\right)$ whilst there is only one hydroxyl ion to every hundred thousand million molecules of water $\left(\frac{1}{10^{11}}\right)$; conversely a solution of washing soda with a pH of 10 has only one hydrogen ion present to every ten thousand million molecules of water $\left(\frac{1}{10^{10}}\right)$ whilst there is a hydroxyl ion present to every ten thousand molecules $\left(\frac{1}{10^4}\right)$.

It is to be noted that the *lower* the pH the *greater* the concentration of H^+ ions and the acidity, whilst the *higher* the pH the *lower* the concentration of H^+ ions and the greater the alkanity.

In the body there is a wide range of pH values, the acid gastric juice having a pH of about 0·8, and the lactic acid of the vagina about 4·5. The blood is on the alkaline side of neutrality with a pH of 7·40, whilst the alkaline pancreatic juice has a high pH of about 8·8.

APPENDIX III

Cell Life

THE CELL

All living plants and animals (including man) have a structure composed essentially of cells and cellular products. The cells which form the human body number many thousands of millions and although their size usually lies between 10μ and 100μ, their individual shape and dimensions differ according to the organ or tissue in which they occur. Thus liver cells, kidney cells, brain cells, etc., have different characteristics dependent on their varying functions and yet they all have basically the same constituents.

Each cell, when it is in its resting stage and is not dividing, consists of a semi-fluid jelly-like material known as protoplasm, which is bounded by a delicate cell membrane. Immersed in it and usually central in position lies a small globule of denser material that stains readily with certain dyes and is known as the nucleus of the cell. The protoplasm that surrounds it is called the cytoplasm.

1. *The cell membrane*. This is a fine pellicle that encloses the cell and acts as a retaining and protective membrane, and at the same time regulates the passage of fluid and dissolved substances in and out of the cell.

2. *The nucleus*. Under the microscope this appears to be a uniform collection of dense stainable material, known as chromatin, but in reality it is composed of separate masses of chromatin immersed in a fluid called nuclear sap or karyoplasm, and enclosed by a fine nuclear membrane. It is this material that forms the chromosomes during cell division. In places there may occur small more darkly staining condensations of chromatin, which are known as nucleoli. Some observers describe a network of threads composed of linin within the nucleus, but this is doubtful. The properties and behaviour of the nucleus during cell division are described below.

3. *The cytoplasm*. This is composed of water in which are present

proteins, fats or lipids, carbohydrates, secretory granules, vacuoles, and dissolved inorganic and organic salts, particularly potassium salts. Also present are certain particles visible under the microscope which are sometimes called the organelles:

(i) A single (sometimes double) small body known as a *centriole*, which is surrounded by a zone of clear cytoplasm to form a centrosome. This lies close to the nucleus and plays a part in the process of cell division, as described later.

(ii) Multiple small structures known as *mitochondria*. These are minute rodlike bodies scattered throughout the cytoplasm which produce energy by a process whereby a substance they contain known as adenosine triphosphate (ATP) changes to adenosine diphosphate (ADP) with the release of energy. It is this energy that enables the cell to carry out its function, such as the muscle cell to contract, the glandular cell to secrete and the nerve cell to transmit an electrical impulse.

(iii) *The Golgi apparatus*. This is a collection of minute rods and granules which form a reticular pattern. Its exact significance is not properly understood, but it is believed to modify cellular secretions.

(iv) *The endoplasmic reticulum*. This is a diffuse network of membranous structure scattered throughout the cytoplasm and only visible under very great magnification. It plays a part in the synthesis of proteins within the cell.

THE PROCESSES OF CELL DIVISION

There are two types of cell division that have to be studied. First, the division that occurs during the normal process of cell growth when a single cell divides into two identical daughter cells—this is known as mitosis or karyokinesis. Secondly, a special form of division occurs in both sexes when the reproductive cells are formed—this is called meiosis.

Mitosis

The process of mitosis by which a cell divides and gives rise to two daughter cells begins with changes in the centrosome and nucleus which lead to splitting of the nucleus into two nuclei, followed by changes in the cytoplasm and cell membrane which result in the production of two new cells. The nuclear changes are described as occurring in four phases:

1. *Prophase*. The centriole if single splits into two centrioles, which separate from each other but remain connected by a star-shaped pattern of radiating filaments in the cytoplasm. At the same time the appearance of the chromatin in the nucleus alters and it becomes revealed as a conglomerate of individual fine threads or filaments known as chromosomes; the nucleoli and nuclear membrane disappear and become incorporated into the pattern of chromosomes. As these changes take place the two centrioles move into position one on each side of the nucleus at opposite poles, and the former star-pattern of fibrils becomes a spindle that extends between them and passes through the cluster of chromosomes.

When the chromosomes are examined under high powers of magnification, each is seen to be composed of two filaments adherent along their lengths and coiled around each other. These are known as chromatids. Each species of animal and plant has its own individual number of chromosomes which is always constant under normal conditions of growth. This is called the diploid number and in the human race is 46. Of this number 44 chromosomes are concerned with growth and development and are called autosomes, whilst two are concerned with sex and are known as the sex chromosomes. Half of the chromosomes have been derived from the original ovum which has given rise to the cell and are thus maternal in origin, and half have come from the original fertilizing spermatozoon and so are paternal in origin.

At one place in each chromosome the chromatids are fused—this point is known as the centromere.

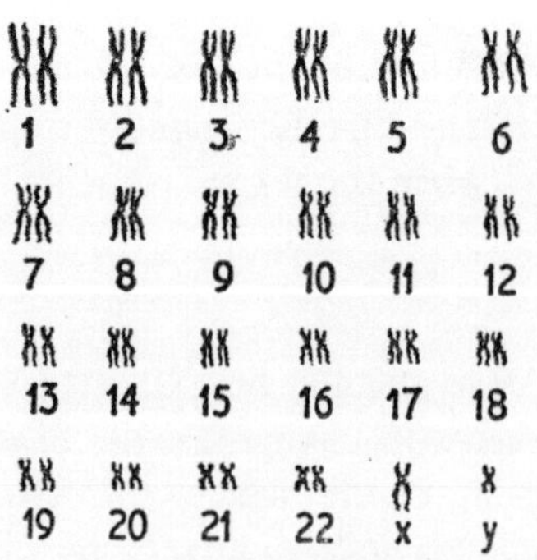

FIGURE 93. Human chromosomes arranged as 22 homologous pairs of autosomes and the X and Y sex chromosomes

It can also be seen that the autosomes occur in pairs, i.e., although they are of different shapes and sizes, with the centromere placed in different positions along their length, each one has an identical fellow with which it becomes paired—these are homologous chromosomes, one of the pair being maternal and the other paternal in origin. Thus in man there are 22 pairs of homologous chromosomes and two sex chromosomes.

Each individual chromosome is composed of a substance called deoxyribonucleic acid (DNA), which is not evenly distributed along the length of the chromosome but occurs in localized nodules, like beads on a string. These are the genes, there being about 2,000 of them present in each autosome. They are responsible for handing on to the daugher cells the qualities and properties of the mother cell. They are thus the locus of heredity.

2. *Metaphase.* The chromosomes become attached in a circle around the equator of the spindle that extends between the two centrioles.

3. *Anaphase.* The centromere of each chromosome splits into two halves and this is followed by the separation of the chromatids along their entire length. Each original chromosome therefore divides longitudinally into too new chromosomes which are identical in structure to each other and to their parent chromosome. These new chromosomes appear to repel each other, and travel in opposite

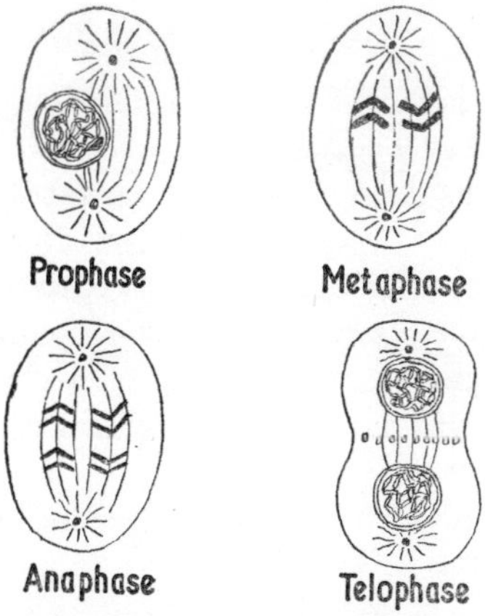

FIGURE 94. Stages of mitosis (only four chromosomes are shown for the sake of clarity)

directions along the threads of the spindle towards the two centrioles. As they approach these bodies they become grouped together, there being the same number of chromosomes in each group as there were chromosomes in the original cell, half still being maternal and the other half paternal in origin.

4. *Telophase.* A nuclear membrane forms around each group of daughter chromosomes as they gradually lose their individuality and merge together to form a new nucleus of each daughter cell. As this forms new nucleoli make their appearance.

Following this splitting of the nucleus, the cell membrane becomes indented around the cell in the plane of cleavage, and the cytoplasm gradually becomes divided into two halves, each of which surrounds one of the new nuclei. The cell membrane then encloses each division of the cytoplasm so that two new daughter cells, each with its nucleus, centrosome, cytoplasm and organelles, and cell membrane have been formed from the original cell. At first each daugher cell is smaller than the original cell, but in the process of normal growth it enlarges so that in due course it becomes identical with its predecessor.

The whole process of mitosis takes about one hour to occur.

Meiosis

This type of cell division occurs in the formation of the reproductive cells or gametes, i.e., the ovum in the female and the spermatozoon in the male. This involves a double type of cleavage:

First Cleavage

(i) *Prophase.* This is similar to the mitotic prophase in that a spindle develops in the usual way between the two centrioles and the chromosomes in homologous pairs become demarcated. However, as each chromosome separates into its two constituent chromatids the homologous chromosomes become coiled closely around each other and chromatin becomes exchanged between them. In this way there is an interchange of genetic material between chromosomes derived from maternal and paternal sources. After this exchange the chromosomes uncoil and separate.

(ii) *Metaphase.* The 23 pairs of chromosomes become attached to the equator of the spindle as in mitosis.

(iii) *Anaphase.* The important distinction from mitosis now occurs. The chromosomes do not divide longitudinally but instead each member of an homologous pair becomes drawn along tbe spindle away from its partner towards one of the two centrioles, so that each daughter nucleus as it is formed contains only 23 chromosomes, i.e., one chromosome of each original pair. This is sometimes called the reduction division.

(iv) *Telophase.* The formation of two new nuclei with their nuclear membranes takes place and this is followed by the division of the cytoplasm and cell membrane.

This new number of chromosomes in the daughter cells (23) is said to be the haploid number in distinction to the original diploid number of 46.

Second Cleavage

(i) *Prophase.* Immediately after the preceding telophase, the nuclear membrane disappears and the changes of prophase are seen again with the formation of the centrioles and spindle.

(ii) *Metaphase.* The 23 chromosomes become attached to the spindle in the usual way.

(iii) *Anaphase.* Each chromosome splits longitudinally as in mitosis, and the separated chromatids pass to opposite poles.

(iv) *Telophase.* This occurs normally, the new nuclei and nuclear membranes being formed in the usual way.

The results of these changes are that four cells have formed from the original cell, the first cleavage producing two cells with the haploid number of chromosomes as a result of the reduction division, and the second cleavage increasing these to four cells. Not only are the chromosomes of these cells half the original number but they also have a different genetic content as a result of the chromatin interchange.

In the human female this process is intimately associated with ovulation and fertilization. In the primordial follicles of the newborn baby the ova, which may be called primary oocytes, have begun the first cleavage of meiosis, but the process goes no further and the nucleus of the cell remains in the prophase state during childhood and does not proceed to metaphase and anaphase. This arrested state is known as the dictyate stage. Immediately preceding ovulation, under the influence of luteinizing hormone, the first cleavage is finally completed, resulting in the halving of the number of chromosomes as described above, one half being cast off as the first polar body and the other half remaining in the ovum, which may now be termed the secondary oocyte. The second cleavage, resulting in the expulsion of the second polar body, only takes place if fertilization occurs (see Figure 45, p. 104).

In the human male spermatozoa are formed from large cells known as spermatogonia in the testicle. These divide into primary spermatocytes containing 46 chromosomes, each of which undergoes meiotic or reduction division into two secondary spermatocytes, containing 23 chromosomes, and then into four spermatids, without the production of any polar bodies. Each spermatid then grows and develops into a spermatozoon with a complement therefore of 23 chromosomes (see Figure 46, p. 104).

It will thus be seen that immediately prior to fertilization, the ovum and the spermatozoon each contains 23 chromosomes.

Fertilization

Following the entry of the spermatozoon into the ovum, the head and neck becomes detached from the middle piece and tail which disappear and are no longer recognizable in the cytoplasm of the ovum. The head of the sperm swells and becomes the male pronucleus, whilst changes of prophase produce the 23 chromosomes. At the same time the nucleus of the ovum completes its second cleavage as already described and becomes the female pronucleus, the second polar body being extruded into the perivitelline space.

Approximation and fusion of the two pronuclei next occur. A centrosome believed to contain the centriole from the sperm, divides and forms the characteristic spindle. The two sets of 23 chromosomes from the two pronuclei arrange themselves around the equator of the spindle as in metaphase in such a way that the corresponding homologous chromosomes lie alongside each other, one coming from the ovum and one from the sperm. The fertilized ovum or zygote now contains the diploid number of 46 chromosomes.

The chromosomes then split in anaphase and are drawn along the spindle to opposite poles in telephase and two daughter cells are produced in the manner already described. This is the first step in segmentation of the zygote, which continues as described in Chapter 5.

THE CHEMICAL STRUCTURE OF CHROMOSOMES

It has already been stated that chromosomes are composed of chromatin, arranged as a succession of genes to form a filament or thread. The chief chemical constituent of chromatin and the genes is a nucleoprotein which contains a type of nucleic acid known as deoxyribonucleic acid (DNA). The cytoplasm of the cell contains a similar substance known as ribonucleic acid (RNA). These are both of outstanding importance to the life and functions of the cell.

DNA has a high molecular weight and the atoms of which the molecules are composed form long chains which wind around each other like a spiral or helix, being connected along their length by transverse bonds. The structure of the molecule is thus like a ladder which is twisted on itself.

The chains winding around each other (corresponding to the sides of the ladder) consists of many sugar (deoxyribose) and phosphate groups joined together, whilst the transverse bonds (corresponding to the rungs) linking them together are composed of four bases joined up in pairs. These bases are adenine, thymine, guanine and cytosine occurring in regular sequence. A unit consisting of a base, sugar and phosphate group is known as a nucleotide, millions of which make up a single chromosome.

The genes manufacture the second form of nucleic acid, RNA, which contains a different sugar (ribose) and an alternative base (uracil). This enters the cytoplasm and there forms proteins and enzymes which are typical of the cell, and thereby confer upon it its qualities and enable it to carry out its functions.

As a result of the double structure of the DNA molecule, it is able to split along its entire length, after which each half can duplicate itself and reform the complete molecule. In this way DNA is able to reproduce and perpetuate itself.

During the process of cell growth and division this property of perpetuation enables the DNA to remain constant during the lifetime of the cell and its descendants. When mitosis occurs the mother cell thus hands on identical genes to each of the daughter cells; during meiosis the qualities of the parent cell inherent in its genes are passed to the reproductive cell, and ultimately to the new individual.

The sequence of nucleotides along the length of the DNA molecular chains varies, and this variation, occurring in different genes, endows each gene with its individual properties. These differences influence the RNA manufactured, and this in its turn produces different proteins and enzymes and so gives rise to the different cells of the body. These differing genes of the chromosomes constitute the genotype of the individual, whilst his resultant physical characteristics comprise his phenotype.

It can be understood that the genes of the chromosomes, through the medium of RNA and the cell proteins and enzymes, control the functions of the cell. When it is remembered that this is occurring in all the millions of cells of the body, and that the genes which control it are derived equally from maternal and paternal sources, the nature of heredity can be appreciated.

SEX CHROMOSOMES

The role of sex chromosomes in determining sex has been described in Chapter 5, but they have additional features of interest. Cells of the female body (apart from the reproductive cells) contain 44 autosomes and two X sex chromosomes. These two X sex chromosomes have been derived from different sources—one has come from the maternal ovum and one from the paternal spermatozoon. Only one of these X chromosomes appears to participate in the normal

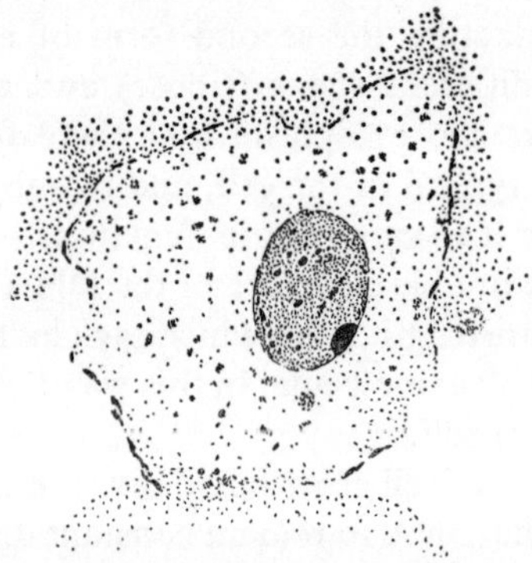

FIGURE 95. Cell showing a Barr body

functioning of the cell, and so disappears within the chromatin mass of the nucleus when the cell is in the resting phase. The other X chromosome remains unchanged and can be seen under favourable circumstances as a black-staining body about 1μ in diameter within the nuclear membrane. It can most easily be identified in certain types of cell such as the squamous cells lining the buccal cavity, when it is referred to as a Barr body. Sometimes, such as in polymorphonuclear leucocytes in the circulating blood, it appears to project through the nuclear membrane into the cytoplasm, when it is termed a 'drumstick'. Examination of these cells from normal individuals, therefore, will reveal the sex to which they belong. If the Barr body or drumstick is present the cell contains two X chromosomes, is said to be chromatin positive, and comes from a female; if there is no Barr body or drumstick in any of the cells visualized then the cell contains only one X chromosome, is said to be chromatin negative, and so comes from a male.

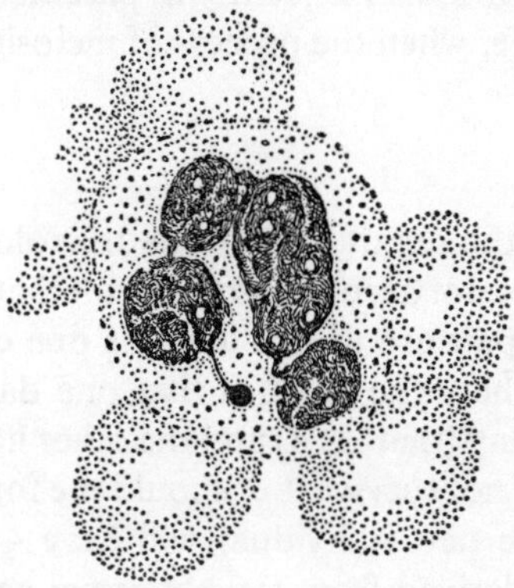

FIGURE 96. Leucocyte showing a 'drumstick'

This procedure is of use in determining the true sex in a case of intersex or hermaphroditism, and is sometimes employed during pregnancy, when the liquor amnii may be tapped and the nuclei of foetal or amniotic cells contained in it will reveal the sex of the foetus.

It has been suggested by Lyon that of the two X chromosomes in each female cell, one has genes that are active and participate in the function of the cell, whilst the other forming the Barr body has inactive genes. Each of these chromosomes may be derived from either maternal or paternal sources—it follows therefore that some cells will have a functioning maternal X chromosome whilst others will have a functioning paternal X chromosome. These cells then may be expected to give rise to different behaviour patterns dependent upon the different origin of their X chromosome. Such differences account for the colour patchiness in the coats of mice and tortoiseshell cats, and also for the absence of a specific enzyme from the red cells of women. This inactivation of one of the X chromosomes in this way is known as Lyonization.

Abnormal Separation of Chromosomes

The process of meiosis involved in the formation of the reproductive cells does not invariably occur in a normal manner. Departure from the normality may occur in many ways, but only those most frequently encountered will now be described. Altogether, however, with the possible exception of Mongolism or Down's syndrome, they are rare. They mostly arise during anaphase, when the chromosomes are splitting and the two halves are being drawn apart towards the centrioles. They occur most frequently in parents towards the end of their reproductive life, when the process of meiosis has lost its vigour and efficiency.

1. *Down's Syndrome*

In this condition the separation of one homologous chromosome pair (number 21) does not occur, with the result that two chromosomes instead of one of a pair are drawn towards one centriole, and none goes towards the other. The result is that one daugher cell has one chromosome too many (that is 24) and the other has one too few (22). The second cell does not survive, but should the former be involved in fertilization then the new individual will have 47 chromosomes in each cell, 24 being derived from the abnormal cell and 23 from the other fertilizing cell. This non-separation of the chromosomes is known as non-disjunction. The individual with 47 chromosomes develops into a patient with Down's syndrome or Mongolism and is said to have trisomy-21. It will be noticed that the sex chromosomes are not involved in this malfunction, so that the syndrome may occur in persons of each sex.

2. *Turner's Syndrome*

In this abnormality the sex chromosomes are affected. Non-disjunction of the two X chromosomes in the ovum similarly occurs so that there are some ova with no X chromosomes and some with two X chromosomes. If fertilization occurs between any X-bearing sperm and the former cell, the new individual will have only 45 chromosomes in each cell of type XO, because one X chromosome from the ovum is missing. This can also result from non-disjunction in the formation of spermatozoa, when a sperm carrying no sex chromosome fertilizes a normal ovum containing a single X chromosome. Such a person has cells that are chromatin negative and is said to be an example of Turner's syndrome or gonadal dysgenesis. The incidence of this condition is about 1 in 2,500 persons.

Such an individual grows up outwardly resembling a female although she has infantile sex organs, inactive 'streak' ovaries, is very short with scanty hirsutes, has a wide 'webbed' neck, a wide carrying angle of the arms (cubitus valgus), and deformities of the ears and digits. These persons always have amenorrhoea and are always sterile.

3. *Superfemale*

These cases also result from non-disjunction, but in this event an ovum containing two X chromosomes as described above is fertilized by an X-bearing spermatozoon, and the resultant individual has three X sex chromosomes and a total complement of 47 chromosomes to the cell. Two Barr's bodies are present in these cases. However, in distinction from what the name suggests, these persons usually grow up with an infantile genital tract, oligomenorrhoea and sterility, and perhaps mental deficiency. The incidence is about 1 in 1,000.

4. *Klinefelter's syndrome*

Another result of non-disjunction may be that a two X-bearing ovum unites with a Y-bearing sperm to produce an individual with

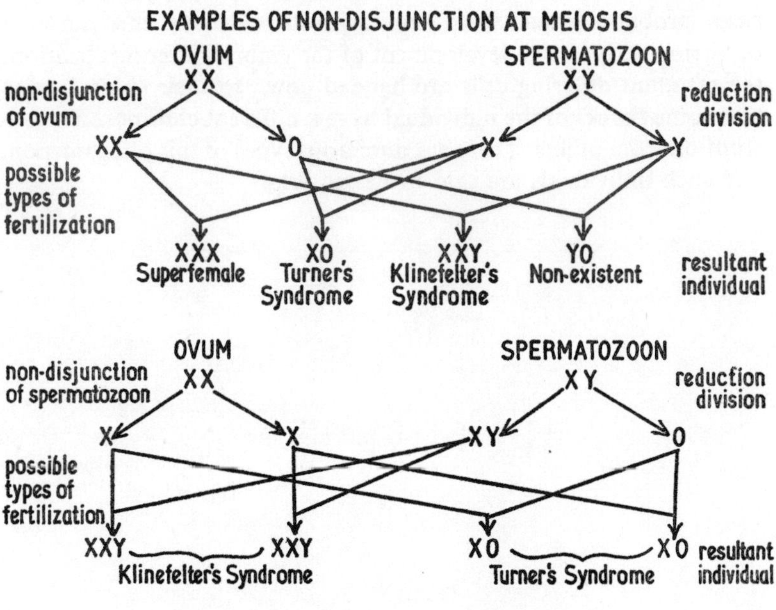

FIGURE 97. Examples of non-disjunction

three sex chromosomes, XXY, and a total of 47. This state of affairs might also result from a normal X-bearing ovum uniting with an XY-bearing sperm. The result is to produce a person who resembles a male (because his cells contain a Y chromosome), but who is chromatin positive (because like a female he has two X chromosomes). Such a person is said to be an example of Klinefelter's syndrome. He is usually tall with infantile testicles, large breasts, and perhaps mental defects, and although he is able to have sexual intercourse he will be sterile. The incidence is about 1 in 500.

5. *Mosaicism*

Abnormalities of development may not occur in such clear-cut clinical entities as the above. Sometimes individuals are seen particularly in cases of intersex, where some abnormal features are present but not all. For example, some individuals show an intermediate state between Turner's syndrome and a normal female, or between the syndrome and a normal male. These persons are likely to have some cells with an XO chromosome pattern and some with the normal XX female pattern or the normal XY male pattern. Such cases probably result from non-disjunction of sex chromosomes occurring early in the development of the embryo after fertilization; the resultant differing cells are handed down to their successors so that some tissues of the individual have a different chromosome constitution from others. There are numerous types of this phenomenon, and such individuals are said to be mosaics.

Index

INDEX

INDEX

INDEX

INDEX

INDEX